Diagnostics of Traditional Chinese Medicine

T0385286

Companion volumes

Basic Theories of Traditional Chinese Medicine
Edited by Zhu Bing and Wang Hongcai
ISBN 978 1 84819 038 2
International Acupuncture Textbooks

Meridians and Acupoints
Edited by Zhu Bing and Wang Hongcai
ISBN 978 1 84819 037 5
International Acupuncture Textbooks

Acupuncture Therapeutics
Edited by Zhu Bing and Wang Hongcai
ISBN 978 1 84819 039 9
International Acupuncture Textbooks

Case Studies from the Medical Records of Leading Chinese Acupuncture Experts
Edited by Zhu Bing and Wang Hongcai
ISBN 978 1 84819 046 7
International Acupuncture Textbooks

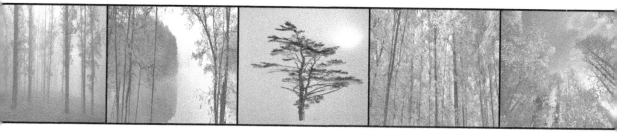

International
Acupucture
Textbooks

Diagnostics of Traditional Chinese Medicine

Chief Editors: Zhu Bing and Wang Hongcai

Advisor: Cheng Xinnong

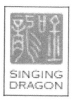

SINGING
DRAGON

London and Philadelphia

China Beijing International Acupuncture Training Center
Institute of Acupuncture and Moxibustion
China Academy of Chinese Medical Sciences
Advisor: Cheng Xinnong
Chief Editors: Zhu Bing, Wang Hongcai
Deputy Editors: Hu Xuehua, Huang Hui, Yu Min, Wang Huizhu
Members of the Editorial Board: Huang Hui, Hong Tao, Hu Xuehua, Liu Xuan, Liu Yuting, Wang Fang, Wang Hongcai, Wang Huizhu, Wang Yue, Wu Mozheng, Yu Min, Zhu Bing, Zhang Nan, Zhang Yi

Copyright © People's Military Medical Press 2008 and 2010

First published in 2010
by Singing Dragon (an imprint of Jessica Kingsley Publishers)
in co-operation with People's Military Medical Press
116 Pentonville Road
London N1 9JB, UK
and
400 Market Street, Suite 400
Philadelphia, PA 19106, USA

Library of Congress Cataloging in Publication Data
A CIP catalog record for this book is available from the Library of Congress

British Library Cataloguing in Publication Data
A CIP catalogue record for this book is available from the British Library

ISBN 978 1 84819 036 8

Printed and bound in the United States

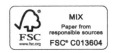

MIX
Paper from
responsible sources
FSC® C013604

CHINA BEIJING INTERNATIONAL ACUPUNCTURE TRAINING CENTER

China Beijing International Acupuncture Training Center (CBIATC) was set up in 1975 at the request of the World Health Organization (WHO) and with the approval of the State Council of the People's Republic of China. Since its foundation, it has been supported and administered by WHO, the Chinese government, the State Administration of Traditional Chinese Medicine (SATCM) and the China Academy of Chinese Medical Sciences (CACMS). Now it has developed into a world-famous, authoritative training organization.

Since 1975, aiming to popularize acupuncture to the world, CBIATC has been working actively to accomplish the task, 'to perfect ways of acupuncture training and provide more opportunities for foreign doctors', assigned by WHO. More than 30 years' experience has created an excellent teaching team led by the academician, Professor Cheng Xinnong, and a group of professors. The multiple courses here are offered in different languages, including English, German, Spanish and Japanese. According to statistics, so far CBIATC has provided training in acupuncture, Tuina Massage, Traditional Chinese Medicine, Qigong, and so on for over 10,000 medical doctors and students from 106 countries and regions.

The teaching programmes of CBIATC include three-month and various short courses, are carefully and rationally worked out based on the individual needs of participants. Characterized by the organic combination of theory with practice, there are more than ten cooperating hospitals for the students to practice in. With professional teaching and advanced services, CBIATC will lead you to the profound and wonderful world of acupuncture.

Official website: www.cbiatc.com
Training support: www.tcmoo.com

PREFACE

More than 2000 years ago, a Chinese doctor named Bianque saved the life of a crown prince simply with an acupuncture needle. The story became one of the earliest acupuncture medical cases and went down in history. It is perhaps since then that people have been fascinated by the mystery of acupuncture and kept on studying it. In 1975, at the request of the World Health Organization, an acupuncture school was founded in Beijing, China, namely the China Beijing International Acupuncture Training Center. As one of the sponsor institutions, the Center compiled a textbook of Chinese Acupuncture and Moxibustion for foreign learners, published in 1980 and reprinted repeatedly afterwards, which has been of profound, far-reaching influence. It has been adopted as a 'model book' for acupuncture education and examination in many countries, and has played a significant role in the global dissemination of acupuncture.

Today, with the purpose of extending this 'authentic and professional' knowledge, we have compiled a series of books entitled *International Acupuncture Textbooks* to introduce incisively the basic theories of Traditional Chinese Medicine (TCM) and acupuncture–moxibustion techniques, by building on and developing the characteristics of the original textbook of Chinese Acupuncture and Moxibustion; and presenting authoritatively the systematic teaching materials with concise explanation based on a core syllabus for TCM professional education in China.

In addition, just as the same plant might have its unique properties when growing in different geographical environments, this set of books may reflect, in its particular style, our experience accumulated over 30 years of international acupuncture training.

Zhu Bing and Wang Hongcai

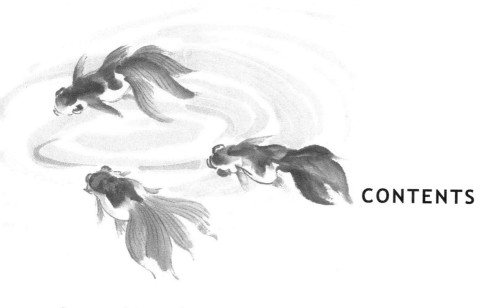

CONTENTS

CHAPTER

INTRODUCTION

1

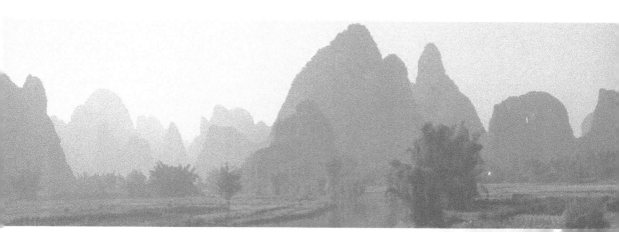

I. THE CONCEPT OF DIAGNOSTICS OF TRADITIONAL CHINESE MEDICINE (TCM)

Guided by the theory of Chinese medicine, the diagnostics of TCM involves studying how to differentiate and diagnose diseases. It is the bridge between the basic theories and treatments, in the system of TCM.

II. THE CONTENT OF DIAGNOSTICS OF TCM

1. DIAGNOSTIC METHODS: INSPECTION, AUSCULTATION AND OLFACTION, INQUIRING, AND PALPATION

1.1 Inspection

Observation by the doctor, using his eyes, of the systemic and regional changes in the patient's vitality, colour, appearance, secretions and excretions.

1.2 Auscultation and olfaction (listening and smelling)

Listening to the patient's speech, respiration, and cough, and smelling the odours of the patient.

1.3 Inquiring

Asking the patient, or the patient's companion, about the conditions associated with the illness in order to understand the pathological process.

1.4 Palpation

Includes feeling the pulse, and palpation of different parts of the patient's body.

2. EIGHT PRINCIPLES

The Eight Principles describe the eight basic categories of syndromes – namely, Yin and Yang, exterior and interior, Cold and Heat, and deficiency and excess – used to analyze the location and nature of diseases, and the relative strength of the pathogenic factors and antipathogenic Qi.

3. SYNDROME DIFFERENTIATION

This involves a comprehensive analysis of the symptoms and signs obtained through applying the four diagnostic methods and interpreting them through the Eight Principles (see Figure 1.1).

Differentiation of syndromes according to the Theory of the Eight Principles Differentiation of syndromes according to the Theory of Aetiology	Applicable for all clinical treatments
Differentiation of syndromes according to the Theory of Qi, Blood and Body Fluid Differentiation of syndromes according to the Theory of the Zang Fu Organs	Applicable for diagnosing endogenous diseases
Differentiation of syndromes according to the Theory of the Six Meridians Differentiation of syndromes according to the Theory of Wei-defence, Qi, Ying-nutrient and Xue-Blood Differentiation of syndromes according to the Theory of the Triple Burner	Applicable for diagnosing acute febrile diseases

Figure 1.1

Each method has its own features and lays stress on a particular aspect while connecting with and supplementing the others.

4. HOW TO WRITE CASE REPORTS

This is the basic skill that should be mastered by clinical doctors.

III. THE PRINCIPLES OF DIAGNOSTICS OF TCM

1. To examine the entirety of the pathological changes and the environmental conditions of the patient.

2. To differentiate the syndromes and seek causative factors.

3. To use the four diagnostic methods in combination for a comprehensive analysis.

DIAGNOSTICS

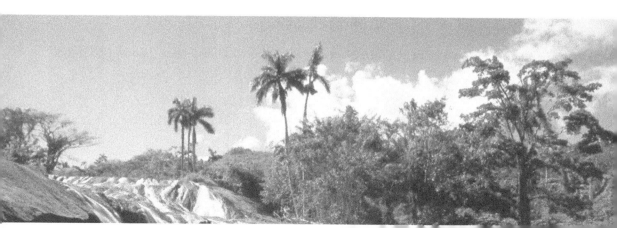

I. INSPECTION

Inspection is aimed at diagnosing through observation of the whole body, including the excreta of the patients, to understand their pathological changes. Inspection includes the observation of vitality, colour, appearance, and so on.

1. OBSERVATION OF VITALITY

Shen (vitality)

Broad meaning: General manifestation of the vital activities of the human body. Shen refers to Life.

Narrow meaning: Spiritual activities. Shen refers to Spirit.

Material basis

Shen comes from the congenital Essence. It depends on the nourishment of acquired Essence after birth and the support of the normal functions of the Zang Fu organs.

The significance of the observation of vitality

To understand the strength of the antipathogenic Qi of the human body and the severity of the disease.

Observation of vitality focuses on the expression of the eye, consciousness and spirit, complexion, and appearance.

With vitality, less vitality, without vitality, false vitality

One can observe four types of vitality.

With vitality: The antipathogenic Qi has not yet been damaged, indicating that the disease is mild.

Less vitality: Here, the antipathogenic Qi is weak, as seen in deficiency patients.

Without vitality: This indicates the critical stage of a disease.

False vitality: A patient with serious disease shows a false manifestation of good vitality, this being the sign of approaching death.

	Manifestations	Significance
With vitality	Normal appearance and colour, lustrous complexion, keen response, a sparkle in the eyes, full consciousness with normal speeches and movements, and regular respiration	Healthy. Even though the patient is diseased, the disease is mild, with a good prognosis
Less vitality	Listlessness, forgetfulness, sleepiness, low voice, tiredness, slow in movement	Weakness of functions of the Zang Fu organs. Mild disease with a good prognosis
Without vitality	Emaciation, with diseased complexion, slow in response, without sparkle in the eyes, not full consciousness, abnormal speech and movements (delirium, involuntary movement of fumbling and picking at the bed or clothes), and respiration	Failure of functions of the Zang Fu organs, poor prognosis
False vitality	Suddenly with flushed cheeks, sparkle in the eyes, and good appetite	Failure of Yin to control Yang causing Yang to float out, showing a false phenomenon of 'getting better', being a critical sign of separation of Yin and Yang and impending death

Abnormal mentality

Depressive mental disorder: Manifested by dejection, reticence or incoherent speech, laughing and crying. Mostly caused by stagnation of Phlegm-Qi misting the Mind.

Manic mental disorder: Manifested by shouting, restlessness and violent behaviours. Mostly caused by excessive Yang disturbing the Mind or Blood stasis misting the Mind.

Epilepsy: Manifested by falling down in a fit, loss of consciousness, foam on the lips, screams, with eyes staring upward, and convulsions. Mostly caused by Liver Wind bringing the Phlegm upward to mist the Mind, or Phlegm Fire disturbing the Heart.

2. OBSERVATION OF COLOUR

The colour and lustre of the face are observed

The colour and lustre of the face are the outward manifestations of the Qi and Blood of the Zang Fu organs, and so the observation of the colour and lustre is helpful in diagnosing.

Discolourations include: blue which suggests Liver disease, red which suggests Heart disease, yellow which suggests Spleen disease, pale which suggests Lung disease, and dark grey which suggests Kidney disease.

The corresponding areas of Zang Fu on the face

People of different races have different skin colours. However, a lustrous skin with natural colour pertaining to the person's Element is considered normal. A normal coloured and lustrous face implies the person is in good health with abundant Qi and Blood, and good function of the Zang Fu organs.

Host colour: Wood people have a complexion tending to blue, Earth people to yellow, Fire people to red, Metal people have a pale complexion, and Water people have a dark grey tinge to the complexion.

Guest colour (according to the season): For example, the face should be slightly blue in spring, slightly red in summer, slightly yellow in late summer, slightly pale in autumn, and somewhat dark grey in winter.

Both host and guest colours are normal physiological phenomena.

Diseased colours: This refers to those whose complexion is too dark or too bright, or whose colour is not changed to reflect changing life conditions.

Normal or abnormal:

- *Normal*: Bright with lustre; mild disease, no failure of Zang Fu organs; still with Stomach-Qi; good prognosis.

- *Abnormal*: Dark and dry; severe disease, failure of Zang Fu organs; exhaustion of Stomach-Qi; poor prognosis.

Plain Questions describes the colours of faces as follows: green like a bird's green feather, red like a cock's-comb, yellow like the belly of a crab, white like lard, and black like the feather of a crow – these are thought to be the alive colours. Green like dead grass, red like stagnated Blood, yellow like the fruit of an unripe lemon, white like a piece of dry bone, and black like coal are dead colours.

Indications of discolorations

Blue face

Manifestations	Significance	
Pale with a blue tinge	Yang deficiency with excessive Yin, invasion of Cold, severe pain, prolonged Liver disease	Cold syndrome, pain syndrome, Blood stasis, infantile convulsions
Grey with purple lips	Failure of Heart Yang, Heart Blood stasis, stagnation of Lung-Qi	
Blue in glabellum and around the nose and mouth of a child	Infantile convulsions	
Grey with Cold extremities	Collapse of Heart Yang	
Blue with red cheeks	Alternation of Cold and Heat	

Red face

Manifestations	Significance	
Red in entire face with fever	Excess Heat syndrome	Fever due to exposure to exogenous pathogenic factors, Heat syndrome, floating Yang syndrome
Flushed cheeks	Yin deficiency with internal Heat	
Severe disease with pale but occasionally red cheeks	Floating Yang syndrome (true Cold with false Heat, critical stage)	

Yellow face

Manifestations		Significance		
Sallow complexion		Qi deficiency of Spleen and Stomach		Spleen deficiency, Damp retention
Sallow and puffy face		Spleen deficiency with retention of Damp		
Entire body including face and eyes is yellow	Bright	Jaundice	Yang jaundice with Damp Heat retention	
	Dark		Yin jaundice with Cold Damp and Blood stasis	
Yellow and grey		Liver-Qi stagnation and Spleen deficiency		

Pale face

Manifestations	Significance	
Pale	Deficiency of Qi and Blood	Deficiency Cold syndrome, Qi and Blood deficiency, loss of blood
Pale and puffy	Yang deficiency with water retention	
Bright white	Collapse of Yang Qi, Yin Cold stagnation, big loss of blood	

Black face

Manifestations	Significance	
Dark grey	Kidney Yang deficiency	Kidney deficiency, Cold syndrome, Blood stasis, fluid retention
Black and withered dry	Exhaustion of Kidney Essence, deficiency Fire consuming Yin	
Dark with scaly skin	Prolonged Blood stasis	
Darkness around eyes	Kidney deficiency with water retention, Cold Damp	

Indications of the five discolourations of the face

Colour	Five Elements	Five Zang	Indications and pathogenesis	Characteristics
Blue	Wood	Liver	*Wind*: Failure of Liver in keeping free flow of Qi, causing obstruction of Blood *Pain*: Obstruction of Qi causing Blood stasis *Cold*: Contraction and stagnation of Cold causing obstruction of Blood *Blood stasis*: Obstruction of meridians	Blue complexion Paroxysmal blue black Blue purple
Red	Fire	Heart	*Heat*: Heat makes the Blood circulation accelerate and the vessels are full of blood Excess Deficiency	Whole face red Flushed cheeks Red face like make-up
Yellow	Earth	Spleen	*Damp*: Damp – retention of Damp, obstruction of Qi and Blood Jaundice – retention of Damp – Yang jaundice/Yin jaundice *Deficiency*: Spleen deficiency – poor production of blood, failure of transportation of Water, obstruction of Qi and Blood	Dusty yellow Orange yellow Smoke yellow Yellowish and skinny Yellowish and puffy
White	Metal	Lung	*Deficiency*: Yang deficiency Qi deficiency Blood deficiency *Blood loss*: Not enough blood in vessels	Pale Pale and yellowish
Black	Water	Kidney	*Cold*: Blood circulation being stagnated *Deficiency*: Yang deficiency Yin deficiency with internal Fire *Fluid retention*: Kidney deficiency causing water retention and obstruction of Qi and Blood *Blood stasis*: Obstruction of meridians	Dark Dark and dry Dark around eyes Purple dark

3. OBSERVATION OF APPEARANCE

This refers to the body shape, movement and posture related to disease.

The functions of the Zang Fu organs, whether normal or not, can be reflected in the body shape, movement and posture of the patient. People with different constitutions have different susceptibility to different diseases and different ways in which the diseases develop. Thus, observation of the appearance is helpful for diagnosing.

The appearance of a patient and its clinical significance

Appearance			Significance
Strong or weak	Strong	Big bones, rich muscles, moistened skin	Strong viscera, ample Qi and Blood, good prognosis
	Weak	Small bones, thin muscles, dry skin	Weak viscera, deficient Qi and Blood, poor prognosis
Obese or skinny	Obese	Overweight, good appetite, strong muscles, vigorous	Big body shape, mostly excess and Heat syndrome
		Overweight, poor appetite, short neck, loose skin, listlessness	Big body shape, deficiency of Qi, mostly Phlegm Damp and Windstroke
	Skinny	Skinny, good appetite	Fire in the Middle Burner, Yin deficiency, susceptible to Xiaoke-diabetes
		Skinny, poor appetite	Weakness of the Middle Burner
		Extremely skinny	Failure of Zang Fu
		Skinny, flushed cheeks, dry skin	Yin deficiency with internal Heat, susceptible to consumptive cough
		Skinny, pale complexion, shortness of breath, inactive in talking	Qi and Blood deficiency
Chicken breast, kyphosis			Congenital deficiency, Kidney deficiency, weakness of the Spleen and Stomach
Drum-like thorax			Retention of fluid and Phlegm in the Lung or failure of the Kidneys in receiving Qi
Ascitis and abdominal distention			Liver-Qi stagnation or Spleen deficiency causing water retention and Blood stasis

Constitution

Constitution	Manifestations	Significance
People with balance of Yin and Yang	Proper body shape, in good health, strong in self-regulation and adaptability	Not susceptible to diseases, or quick in recovery
People with excessive Yin	Obese, not active in movement, easily tired, aversion to cold, preference for heat	Excessive Yin with deficient Yang
People with excessive Yang	Skinny, not active in movement, hot temper, aversion to heat, preference for cold	Excessive Yang with deficient Yin

The posture of the patient

Active, supine, extension: Yang, Heat, Excess syndromes.

Inactive, prone, curved: Yin, Cold, Deficiency syndromes.

Lying facing outwards, free in turning the body, restless in bed: Yang, Heat, Excess syndromes.

Lying facing the wall, difficulty in turning the body, not active in movement: Yin, Cold, Deficiency syndromes.

	Manifestations	Clinical significance
Sitting	Sitting with prone position	Lung deficiency with less Qi
	Sitting with supine position	Lung excess with Qi going upward
	Sitting with difficulties in respiration	Cough with asthmatic breathing, or retention of water in chest and abdomen
Lying	Supine with legs stretched out and blanket removed	Excess Heat syndrome
	Curved in bed and covered heavily with blanket	Deficiency Cold syndrome
	Lying only, sitting causing dizziness	Qi and Blood deficiency

	Manifestations	Clinical significance
Abnormal movement	Convulsion, opisthotonus	Extreme Heat producing Wind, or infantile convulsions
	Fingers and toes trembling	Yin deficiency stirring up Wind
	Weakness of arms and legs with muscular atrophy	Wei syndrome
	Joint pain with difficulties in movement	Bi syndrome
	Paralysis of limbs with numbness, or spasm of limbs	Paralysis
	Falling down in a fit with loss of consciousness, hemiplegia, deviation of mouth and eyes	Windstroke with Zang Fu being attacked
	Clear consciousness, hemiplegia, or only deviation of mouth and eyes	Windstroke with meridians and collaterals being attacked
	Falling down in a fit with loss of consciousness, mouth agape, hands open, incontinence of urine	Flaccid syndrome of Windstroke
	Clenched jaws, tightly closed hands	Tense syndrome of Windstroke
	Falling down in a fit but with normal respiration	Jue syndrome

4. OBSERVATION OF THE HEAD AND FIVE SENSE ORGANS

According to the Theory of Zang Xiang (viscera image), the sense organs and orifices are connected with the internal organs. They are the canals connecting the inside of the body with the outside.

4.1 Observation of the head and face

	Manifestations	Significance
Shape of head	Macrocrania	Congenital Kidney Essence deficiency with Water stagnated in the crania
	Microcrania	Congenital Kidney Essence deficiency with maldevelopment of the crania
	Squared skull	Kidney Essence deficiency or Spleen and Stomach deficiency with maldevelopment of the crania
Fontanel	Bulging of the fontanel	Excess Heat syndrome – Fire attacking upward, or Wind Heat, Damp Heat causing the diseased brain
	Sunken fontanel	Deficiency syndrome – Body Fluid damaged by vomiting and diarrhoea, Qi and Blood deficiency, congenital Kidney Essence deficiency causing inadequate filling of the brain
	Metopism	Kidney-Qi deficiency with maldevelopment of the crania
Shaking of head	Involuntary shaking of head	Liver Wind stirring up, Qi and Blood deficiency due to old age
Swelling of face	Yang oedema (quick onset, starting from eyelids)	Oedema – dysfunction of Lung, Spleen and Kidney, retention of water flowing to the skin
	Yin oedema (slow onset, starting from lower limbs)	
	Erysipelas on head (red swelling skin with pain)	Wind Fire – toxin attacking upward
	Infection with swollen head (flushed swollen face with sore throat)	Epidemic pathogenic factor causing Fire-toxin attacking upward
Cheek swelling	Mumps (sudden onset of cheek swelling with sore throat and poor hearing)	Virulent Heat pathogen
Deviation of eye and mouth	Windstroke with meridians and collaterals being attacked (failure of chewing and speaking)	Meridians and collaterals being attacked by Wind, Wind and Phlegm retention

4.2 Observation of the neck

	Manifestations	Significance
Goitre	The mass moving with swallowing	Liver-Qi stagnation, Phlegm retention
Scrofula	Bean-sized masses like stringed pearls	Yin deficiency of Lung and Kidney, deficiency Fire condensing Body Fluid resulting in Phlegm retention, Fire-toxin causing Qi and Blood stagnation causing Phlegm to block the neck region
Stiffness and softness of neck	Stiffness of head	Excessive pathogenic factor – Fire attacking
	Softness of head, heaviness of head	Deficient antipathogenic Qi – Kidney-Qi deficiency
Vessels abnormality	Jumping of vessels	Oedema
	Venous engorgement	Failure of Heart Yang, attack of the Heart by retained fluid

4.3 Observation of the hair

		Manifestations	Significance
Adult	Lustre	Dry, sparse, falling out	Essence and Blood deficiency
		White at a young age, accompanied by symptoms of Kidney deficiency	Kidney deficiency
		White at a young age and accompanied by symptoms of Heart deficiency	Exhaustion of Blood due to hard work
	Hair falling	Alopecia areata	Blood deficiency with Wind attack
		Vertex calvities	Exhaustion of Blood due to hard work
		Sparse hair at a young age, accompanied with forgetfulness and lumbar soreness	Kidney deficiency
		Hair falling out, itching with dandruff, oily hair	Blood Heat transformed into dryness, accompanied with Phlegm Damp
Infant	Infantile malnutrition (dry and yellow hair without lustre)		Congenital deficiency, Spleen and Stomach deficiency
	Soft and sparse hair, slow growing		Deficiency of Kidney Essence, or Qi and Blood deficiency

4.4 Observation of the eye

The eye is the opening of the Liver. The essential Qi of all Zang Fu organs pours upward to nourish the eyes.

The Theory of Five Wheels

Eye part	**Pupil**	**Black part**	**Canthus**	**White part**	**Eyelids**
Wheels	Water wheel	Wind wheel	Blood wheel	Qi wheel	Muscle wheel
Zang organ	Kidneys	Liver	Heart	Lungs	Spleen

Indications of diseased colour, appearance and movement

	Manifestations	Significance	
Colour	Redness, swelling and pain of the eye	Excess Heat syndrome	
	White part becoming yellow	Jaundice	
	Pale canthus	Blood deficiency	
	Dark eyelids	Kidney deficiency	
Appearance	Puffy eyelids	Oedema	
	Sunken eyes	Exhaustion of Body Fluid; deficiency of Qi and Blood	
	Exophthalmos with asthmatic breathing	Lung distention	
	Swelling neck with exophthalmos	Goitre	
	Grain-like nodule on the margin of eyelid with slight redness and swelling	Stye	Wind Heat; Fire-toxin from the accumulation of Heat in Spleen and Stomach attacking the eyes
	Diffuse swelling of eyelids with serious redness and swelling	Suppurative blepharitis	
Movement	Contracted pupil	Poisoning, Windstroke due to cerebral haemorrhage	
	Mydriasis	Injury of brain; Windstroke due to cerebral haemorrhage; bluish glaucoma; drug poisoning	
	Staring with loss of consciousness	Fading of essential Qi of Zang Fu organs (critical)	
	Staring upward; looking sideways	Liver Wind stirring upward (critical)	
	Infant sleeping with eyes not completely closed	Deficiency of Spleen-Qi; Qi and Blood deficiency	
	Ptosis	Both eyes	Congenital deficiency, Spleen and Kidney deficiency
		One eye	Spleen-Qi deficiency; Windstroke; cranial diseases; traumatic injury

4.5 Observation of the ear

The ear is the opening of the Kidneys. The Shaoyang Meridians of Hand and Foot go around and into the ear.

Colour, appearance and secretion of the ear

	Manifestations		Significance	
Colour	Thin and dry auricle		Congenital Kidney Yin deficiency	
	White		Cold	
	Black	Blue and black	Pain	
		Dry and withered auricle in burnt black	Consumption of Kidney Essence in a critical condition	
	Red	Swelling	Shaoyang ministerial Fire flaring up	
		Papilla on the back of ear, Cold auricular root	Aurae of measles	
Appearance	Thin auricle		Congenital Kidney-Qi deficiency	
	Auricular atrophy		Exhaustion of Kidney-Qi	
	Scaly dry skin		Prolonged condition of skin with Blood stasis	
	Nodules of external auditory meatus, ear polyp		Stagnation of Liver Fire, ministerial Fire and Stomach Fire	
	Purulent discharge		Infection	Damp Heat of Liver and Gallbladder, Kidney Yin deficiency, flaring up of deficiency Fire
	Swelling and pain in the auditory canal and pulling pain of the auricle		Auditory disease	

4.6 Observation of the nose

The nose is the opening of the Lungs. Pertaining to the Spleen Meridian, the nose is related to the Stomach Meridian of the Foot Yangming Meridian.

Colour, appearance and movement of the nose

	Manifestations	Significance
Colour	Blue of the tip of the nose	Pain in abdomen
	Yellow of the tip of the nose	Damp Heat in the inside
	White of the tip of the nose	Bleeding
	Red of the tip of the nose	Heat in the Lung and Spleen Meridians
	Dry and black nose	Evil Heat sinking
Appearance	Swelling of the tip of the nose with sores	Blood Heat
	Rosacea	Blood Heat entering the Lungs
	Ulceration of bridge of the nose	Syphilis
	Collapse of bridge of the nose, falling of the eyebrow	Lepra
Movement	Flaring of nares	Retention of Phlegm Heat in the Lungs, asthma, Qi deficiency of the Lungs and Kidneys due to prolonged disease
	Running nose	Invasion of Wind and Cold, deficiency of Yang Qi
	Turbid discharge	Retention of Heat in the Lungs and Stomach, invasion of Wind and Heat
	Rhinorrhoea with turbid discharge	Invasion of Wind and Heat, Damp Heat of Liver and Gallbladder
	Epistaxis	Retention of Heat in the Lungs and Stomach, dryness of the Lungs due to Yin deficiency

4.7 Observation of the lips

The Spleen opens into the mouth and is manifested on the lips. The Stomach Meridian goes around the lips.

Colour, appearance and movement of the lips

	Manifestations	Significance
Colour	Rosy lips	Ample Stomach-Qi, harmoniousness of Qi and Blood
	Pale	Blood deficiency
	Light red	Deficiency and Cold. Blood deficiency, Qi deficiency
	Dark red	Excess and Heat
	Blue black	Pain
	Dark purple	Stagnated Heat in the inside
	Blue black lips and mouth	Extreme Cold
	Black around the mouth	Failure of the Kidneys
Appearance	Dry and cracked lips	Heat damaging the Body Fluid
	Salivation	Spleen deficiency with excessive Damp, Windstroke with deviated mouth
	Aphthous stomatitis	Accumulated Heat of the Spleen and Stomach steaming upward
	Thrush	Fetal Heat accumulated in the Heart and Spleen
	Aphthae in children	Accumulated Heat of the Heart and Spleen steaming upward
	Grey spots appearing on the buccal mucosa with blushes around (measles mucous patch)	Aurae of measles
Movement	Lockjaw of the newborn	Qifeng (umbilical Wind) of the newborn
	Mouth agape	Deficiency
	Angular pulling twisting	Stirring of Wind
	Angular deviation	Wind Phlegm blocked in meridians
	Lip Wind (itching, redness, swelling and fluid flowing out from the cracks of lips with a burning pain)	Yangming Fire flaring up
	Carcinoma of lip (cocoon-like hard nodule of the lip causing difficulties in eating)	Accumulated Heat of the Stomach combined with Phlegm stagnating in the lip

4.8 Observation of the teeth and gums

The teeth are the tips of the bones, which are dominated by the Kidneys. The Hand and Foot Yangming Meridians enter the gum.

	Manifestations	Significance
Teeth	Yellow and dry	The Body Fluid damaged by excessive Heat
	Smooth and dry teeth like stone	Excessive Heat of Yangming
	Dried bone-like teeth	Kidney Yin dried up
	Gnashing teeth	Damp Heat stirring up the Wind, convulsive disease
	Clenched jaws	Wind Phlegm stagnated in the meridians, extreme Heat producing Wind
	Grinding teeth in sleep	Internal Heat
	Loose teeth with the roots exposed	Kidney deficiency, deficient Fire flaring up
Gums	Pale	Blood deficiency
	Pale and atrophied	Stomach Yin deficiency, Kidney-Qi deficiency
	Red and swelling	Stomach Fire flaring up
	Bleeding, swelling and pain	Stomach Heat damaging the collaterals
	Bleeding and slightly swelling	Qi deficiency, Kidney Fire damaging the collaterals

4.9 Observation of the throat

The throat is the door of the Lungs and Stomach, and the passage for respiration and swallowing. Many diseases can be detected from the throat, especially those of the Lungs, Stomach and Kidneys.

Colour, appearance and movement of the throat

	Manifestations	Significance
Redness, swelling, ulceration	Redness, swelling and pain with yellow and white purulent spots (tonsillitis)	Accumulated evil Heat of the Lungs and Stomach
	Delicate red throat without serious swelling and pain	Kidney Yin deficiency, deficient Fire flaring up
	Red throat with serious swelling	Accumulated evil Heat of the Lungs and Stomach
	Slightly red throat with diffuse swelling	Phlegm Damp accumulation
	Itching throat with dry cough, slightly red sore throat without swelling	Qi and Yin deficiency, deficiency Fire flaring up
	Rot of throat with redness and swelling around	Excess syndrome
	Prolonged rot, slightly red or pale	Deficiency syndrome
Pseudo-membrane	Loose pseudomembrane easily removed	Stomach Heat, mild disease
	Strong pseudomembrane not easily removed or with rapid recurrence	Evil Heat of the Lungs and Stomach damaging Yin, serious disease
Pus	Swelling with a soft and Water wave-like sensation	Pus formed
	Swelling with a hard and Water wave-like sensation	Pus not yet formed
	Thick and yellow pus	Excess syndrome
	Thin pus with a dirty look	Antipathogenic Qi deficiency, pathogenic Qi excess
	Pus easily discharged, quick healing	Antipathogenic Qi strong
	Pus not easily discharged, slow healing	Antipathogenic Qi weak

4.10 Observation of the external genitalia and anus

The external genitalia, with which the Liver and Gallbladder Meridians connect and around which they go, is the confluence of tendons and the confluence of Taiyin and Yangming, closely relating to the Liver, Gallbladder, Kidneys, Bladder, Taiyin, Shaoyin, Jueyin, Shaoyang and Yangming Meridians. The anus leads to the rectum and Large Intestine, relating to the Lungs, Spleen and Stomach. Both anterior and posterior orifices are closely related with the Ren-Conception and Du-Governor vessels.

	Manifestations	Significance
Anterior orifice	Swelling of the scrotum without itching and pain	Serious oedema
	Transparent swelling of the scrotum (hydrocele)	Liver stagnation, invasion of Cold, Damp Heat, Qi deficiency, long time standing and walking
	Swelling of the scrotum, not transparent, not hard (inguinal hernia)	
	Flaccid constriction of penis (contraction of the external genitalia into the abdomen)	Cold stagnated in the meridians and collaterals, a critical sign of Yin and Yang extreme deficiency
	Prolapse of uterus	Sinking of Qi of Middle Burner, Spleen deficiency
	Sores with fluid flowing	Syphilis
	Infantile scrotum tenesmus or white in colour	Qi and Blood deficiency, weak constitution
Posterior orifice	Fissure of anus with pain and bleeding	Accumulated Heat of Large Intestine, haemorrhoid
	Haemorrhoid	Intestinal Damp Heat, Blood Heat and intestinal dryness, Blood stasis in the anus region
	Anal fistula	
	Prolapse of rectum	Sinking of Qi of Middle Burner, Qi deficiency

4.11 Observation of the skin

A. Colour and moisture of the skin

		Manifestations	Significance
Red		Dark pink in colour (erysipelas)	Heart Fire, Wind Heat or Damp Heat transformed into Fire, combination of Heat and toxins, Blood Heat excess
		Erysipelas moving from one place to another and with swelling and pain	
Yellow	Jaundice	Yang yellow (bright orange, accompanied with yellow sweats and dark yellow urine, thirst, yellow sticky tongue-coating)	Damp Heat of Spleen and Stomach
		Yin yellow (dark smoking, accompanied with aversion to cold, tastelessness, white sticky tongue-coating)	Cold Damp affecting the Spleen and Stomach
Black		Blackish jaundice (yellow blackish dark skin)	Developed from jaundice and caused by excessive sexual activities
Dryness / moisture	Moistened skin		Body Fluid not yet damaged, Blood not deficient
	Dry skin		Body Fluid damaged, Blood deficiency
	Scaled skin	Accompanied with blackness around eyes	Blood stasis
		Accompanied with acute abdominal pain	Abscess

B. Swelling of the skin

Oedema: A depression does not recover quickly if pressed.

Emphysema: A depression does recover quickly if pressed.

		Manifestations	Significance
Oedema	*Yang oedema*	Starts from the head and face and moves to the body	Invasion of exogenous Wind causing the Lungs to fail in dispersing and descending
	Yin oedema	Starts from feet and moves to the body	Spleen and Kidney Yang deficiency with failure to circulate Water causing the retention of Damp
Emphysema		Puffy skin with depression quickly disappeared	Qi stagnation

C. Macule and rash

Macule: Red in colour, not higher than skin.

Rash: Higher than skin.

Macule

	Manifestations		Accompanying symptoms	Significance
Yang macule	Red, scattered, starts from chest and abdominal regions and then moving out to extremities	Fever is over and cleared minded, indicating the pathogenic factors dispelled. It is a mild case	Fever with red face, restlessness and rapid pulse	Heat stagnated in the Lungs and Stomach and Blood Heat penetrating to skin. It is exogenous febrile disease
		High fever with unconsciousness, indicating the pathogenic factors deeply stagnated. It is a serious case		
Yin macule	Light red or dark purple, different sizes, hidden and scattered, started from here or there, coming and going		Pale complexion, looking tired, pale tongue, weak pulse, cold limbs	Qi and Blood deficiency. It is endogenous disease

Rash

	Manifestations	Accompanying symptoms	Significance
Measles	From head and face to chest and abdomen, pink red, millet shaped, getting gradually dense	Coughing, sneezing, running nose and running tears, red threads behind ear, measles appearing with 3–4 days' fever	Invasion of measles virus
	Measles completely appeared, in red colour, disappeared in the order of appearing, fever stopped		Normal development of disease
	High fever, measles do not completely appear, in light red or dark or purple or white. If the measles suddenly disappear and the patient is unconscious, it indicates the measles toxins are going deeply inside		Abnormal development of disease
Rubella	Small, scattered, slightly higher than skin, light red, itching, more in face and neck regions, without desquamation after disappearing of rubella	Low fever or without fever	Invasion of Wind Heat
Urticaria	Itching, slightly red or white rashes merged in patches if scratched, higher than skin, appearing and disappearing		Blood deficiency, meridians and collaterals being attached by Wind, or allergic to certain materials

D. Miliaria alba and varicella

	Manifestations	Significance
Miliaria alba	Small white crystal-like granules, higher than skin, fluid inside, mostly appearing on neck, chest and abdominal regions, with desquamation when disappearing. Accompanied with low fever, fullness in chest and epigastric region, yellow and sticky tongue-coating	Exogenous pathogenic Damp Heat stagnated in skin, seen in summer Heat Damp, and Damp febrile diseases
Varicella	Ellipse, thin fluid inside, crystal-like blisters, without umbilicus on top, in different sizes, appearing in batches, no thick crust formed, no marks left. Accompanied with slight aversion to cold, fever	Invasion of seasonal pathogenic factors on the Spleen and Lung Meridians, transmitting among children
Hot Qi sores	In clusters, millet-like blisters, burning itching, mostly appearing at corner of mouth, eyelids and perineum	Wind Heat blocking in the Lung and Stomach Meridians, seen in high fever patients
Eczema	First in red patches, then quickly swelling, papule with blisters, fluid coming out when broken, scab formation, marks left but later disappear	Wind Damp Heat stagnated in skin, Blood deficiency due to prolonged disease exhausting the Blood and transformed into dryness, thus skin lacks nourishment
Herpes zoster	First burning pain, then clustered blisters with reddish skin around	Liver Fire stirring causing Damp Heat that steams the skin

E. Carbuncles, cellulitis, nail-like boils and furuncles

	Manifestations	Significance
Carbuncle	Red, swelling, with tight root and burning pain *Characteristics*: Yang syndrome, pus formation, easily broken, thick pus, easy healing	Damp Heat and Fire retention, Qi and Blood stagnation, flesh rot
Cellulitis	Diffuse swelling, without change of skin colour, no Heat feeling, no pain *Characteristics*: Yin syndrome, not easily broken, thin pus, not easy healing	Qi and Blood deficiency, Cold Phlegm stagnation, Wind Heat affecting the muscles and sinking into tendons and bones
Nail-like boil	Millet-like boil with hard root, itching, white top, painful *Characteristics*: Appearing on face and hands and feet, sinking of pathogenic factors, easily transmitting	Wind Heat toxins affecting skin with Qi and Blood stagnation in meridians and collaterals
	Red thread-like boil present from distal to proximal region *Characteristics*: Red streaked infection	Evil Heat stagnated inside
Furuncle	Starting from superficial region, small, round, without serious redness, swelling and pain *Characteristics*: Easily broken, then quick healing	Summer Heat and Damp stagnated in skin, internal Damp Heat affecting the superficial part of body, Qi and Blood obstruction

4.12 Observation of the blood vessels in young children

A. Observation of the superficial venules on the palmar side of the index finger of children less than 3 years old

As is the case with the Cunkou pulse in adults, the radial side of the index finger of children pertains to the Lung Meridian of Hand Taiyin, and it is therefore observed for diagnosis. Observation of the superficial venules on the palmar side of the proximal segment of index finger is applicable for children under 3 years old.

Three guan-passes:

- *Wind pass*: The superficial venules on the palmar side of the proximal segment of the index finger.

- *Qi pass*: The superficial venules on the palmar side of the middle segment of the index finger.

- *Life pass*: The superficial venules on the palmar side of the distal segment of the index finger.

B. How to observe

The infant is carried facing towards the light. The doctor holds the index finger of the infant with the left hand and pushes from the life pass to the Qi and Wind passes with the thumb of the right hand with the correct pressure several times to make the venules clearer for observation.

C. What to observe

	Manifestations	Significance
Normal venules	In light red colour and with red yellow concurrence, as long as within the Wind pass, not too exposed, in the shape of oblique and single branch, not thick or thin, becoming shorter and shorter as the child becomes older	
Depth	Exposed	Exterior syndrome
	Deep	Exterior and endogenous syndromes
Colour	Dark	Serious disease
	Light	Mild disease
	Pale	Deficiency
	Stagnated	Excess
	Purple red	Internal Heat
	Fresh red	Exterior syndrome
	Blue	Wind syndrome, pain syndrome
	Purple black	Blood stagnation in critical condition
Shape	Growing longer	Becoming worse
	Growing shorter	Getting relieved
	Becoming thicker	Heat syndrome, Excess syndrome
	Becoming thinner	Cold syndrome, Deficiency syndrome
Length	To Wind pass	Mild disease with pathogens on the superficial
	To Qi pass	Serious disease with pathogens going deep
	To life pass	Critical condition with pathogens going deep into Zang Fu
	Extending through three passes toward the nail	Critical condition with a poor prognosis

4.13 Observation of nails

	Manifestations	Significance
Normal nails	Red, strong, shaped arc, lustrous, the blood colour immediately restored when the pressure is removed	
Colour	Deep red	Heat in the Qi system
	Yellow	Jaundice
	Whitish	Blood deficiency
	Pale	Deficiency Cold
	Black	Blood stasis
	Blue	Cold
Appearance	With pressure, the nail becomes pale, the blood colour restores slowly when the pressure is removed.	Blood stasis, Qi stagnation
	With pressure, the nail becomes pale, the blood colour fails to restore after the pressure is removed.	Blood deficiency
	Flat or depressed	Liver Blood deficiency

4.14 Observation of excreta and secretions
Excreta and secretions

These are the products of the functional activities of the Zang Fu organs. When the Zang Fu organs are diseased, abnormal changes in excreta and secretions will be seen. Sputum and vomit are the products of dysfunctions of the Zang Fu organs. The location and nature of a disease can be judged through observation of excreta and secretions.

Manifestations and significance:

- *White or pale, thinner:* Cold syndrome, Deficiency syndrome.
- *Yellow or dark, thicker:* Heat syndrome, Excess syndrome.

Observation of sputum, saliva, spittle and nasal discharge

	Manifestations	Significance
Sputum	Yellow and thick	Heat sputum – pathogenic Heat consumes Body Fluid
	White and thin	Cold sputum – pathogenic Cold consumes Yang Qi which fails to produce Body Fluid
	Thin with foam	Wind sputum – Liver Wind brings sputum up to disturb the brain, resulting in the accompanying symptoms of dizziness, fullness in chest and asthmatic breathing
	White, large quantity, easy to be spat out	Damp sputum – Spleen deficiency causes the failure to dissolve Damp
	Small quantity, difficult to be spat out	Dry sputum – damage of the Lungs caused by autumn dryness
	Bloody sputum	Heat burns the collaterals of Lungs
	Purulent and bloody sputum	Heat toxins accumulates in the Lungs
Saliva	Cough with spitting of saliva, with mouth agape and shortness of breath	Consumptive Lung disease
	Thin saliva	Spleen and Stomach deficiency Cold, failure of Qi to control Body Fluid
	Saliva flowing without control	Spleen deficiency with failure to control Body Fluid
	Sticky saliva	Damp Heat of Spleen and Stomach, Damp turbidity going upward
Spittle	Large quantity	Stomach Cold, Cold accumulation, Damp stagnation, food retention, Kidney deficiency
Nasal discharge	Turbid discharge	Invasion of Wind Heat
	Clear discharge	Invasion of Wind Cold
	Turbid discharge running	Rhinorrhoea

Observation of vomitus

Manifestations	Accompanied symptoms	Significance
Thin without bad smell	Cold pain in epigastric region	Cold vomiting – Stomach Yang insufficiency; Spleen and Kidney Yang deficiency, invasion of Stomach by Cold
Dirty with sour smell	Burning feeling in epigastric region, thirst	Heat vomiting – Heat affecting the Stomach, Liver Fire affecting the Stomach
Vomit with sour smell and undigested food in it	Distending pain in epigastric region, made worse by pressure	Retention of food in the Stomach
Vomit with undigested food in it	Dull pain in epigastric region, relieved by pressure, pale tongue, weak pulse	Deficiency Cold of Spleen and Stomach
Watery vomit	Feeling dry in mouth but without a desire to drink, sticky tongue-coating, fullness in chest, water sound in Stomach	Fluid retention in Stomach
Yellow green, bitter watery vomit	Distention in hypochondriac region	Damp Heat of Liver and Gallbladder affecting the Stomach
Fresh red, bloody vomit with dark purple pieces and food residue in it	Burning pain in epigastric and hypochondriac regions, red tongue with yellow coating	Accumulated Heat in the Stomach, Liver Fire affecting the Stomach, accumulated Blood in the Stomach

Observation of faeces

	Manifestations	Accompanied symptoms	Significance
Loose stools	Watery stools	Abdominal distention or Cold pain	Cold Damp diarrhoea – invasion of exogenous pathogenic Cold Damp, intake of Cold and raw food causing the failure of Spleen in transportation and transformation
	Stools like minced meat	Mental restlessness, thirst, burning feeling in the anus	Damp Heat diarrhoea – invasion of summer Heat and Damp, intake of unclean food causing the failure of Spleen in transportation and transformation
	With undigested food in it	Abdominal distention, poor appetite, Cold extremities	Spleen (and Kidney) deficiency, diarrhoea – Qi deficiency of Spleen and Stomach or Spleen and Kidney Yang deficiency with the failure of Spleen in transportation and transformation
	Purulent and bloody stools	Abdominal pain with tenesmus	Dysentery – Damp Heat accumulated in the Large Intestine causing its disorders of transportation
	Grey stools, loose or dry	Yellow body and eyes	Jaundice – disorders of Liver and Gallbladder in free flowing of Qi
Dry stools	Constipation	Abdominal distention, dry throat, red tongue without moisture	Intestinal dryness causing the failure of transportation of wastes
Bloody stools	Fresh red Blood on stools or drop of Blood before or after stools		Close Blood – intestine Wind, anal fissure, haemorrhoid
	Dark Blood mixed with stools or asphalt-like stools		Excessive Heat of the Stomach and intestines, failure of the Spleen in controlling Blood

Observation of urine

Manifestations	Significance
Clear, increased volume	Yang deficiency with the failure of Qi to dissolve fluid
Yellow, decreased volume	Heat consuming fluid, sweat, vomiting and diarrhoea consuming fluid
Bloody	Heat damaging collaterals, failure of Spleen and Kidneys in controlling, Damp Heat accumulation in Bladder
Sandy	Prolonged Damp Heat condensing urine
Turbid	Kidney-Qi deficiency with failure in controlling, Damp Heat in the Lower Burner with failure of Qi activities in separating the turbid from the clear

5. OBSERVATION OF THE TONGUE

The tongue is an organ formed of muscle, blood vessels and nerves. The changes in the shape and colour and lustre of the fungiform on the tongue lead to changes in the tongue proper.

The tongue-coating is a layer like moss over the tongue surface. The filiform papillae on the surface and back of tongue relates to changes in tongue-coating. Through meridians and collaterals, the tongue directly or indirectly connects with many Zang Fu organs, especially the Heart, Spleen and Stomach. Because it is the mirror of the Heart, the outward manifestation of the Spleen and its coating is the moss-like layer formed by the steaming of Stomach-Qi. The manifestations on the tongue are closely related to the condition of Qi, Blood and Body Fluid and their circulation.

The tip of the tongue reveals the pathological changes of the Heart and Lungs; its border reveals those of the Liver and Gallbladder; its central part reveals those of the Spleen and Stomach; and its root reveals those of the Kidneys.

Precautions in tongue diagnosis

The tongue should be observed in direct natural light, in the order of coating to the tongue proper and from tip to root. The patient is required to be in a sitting or supine position and protrude his tongue naturally. Some food and drugs may colour the tongue-coating and attention should be paid to the exclusion of false phenomena induced by such factors.

With seasonal changes, the tongue may have slight changes. For instance, the coating is thicker in summer because of the Damp excess and it is thinner and dry in autumn because of seasonal dryness. Age and constitution are also important factors that need to be paid attention to. Cracks on the tongue are often seen in old people, the tongue of fat people is usually bigger and paler, while it is often thinner and red in slim people.

Observation of the thickness and moisture of the tongue-coating and whether it is easily removed by scraping or not is helpful for diagnosis. For example, Damp is predominant in summer, and the tongue-coating is usually thick. Dryness is prevalent in autumn, and the tongue-coating then is mostly thin and dry.

A normal tongue is of proper size, soft in quality, free in movement, slightly red in colour and with a thin layer of white coating that is neither dry nor over moist.

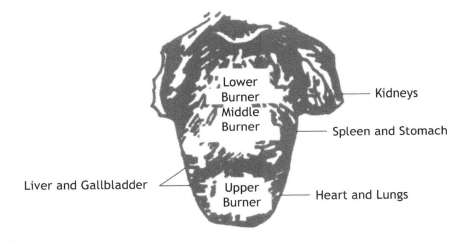

Figure 2.1

What to observe

Tongue proper: Vitality, colour, appearance, movement, reflecting the conditions of the Zang Fu organs, Qi and Blood.

Tongue-coating: Quality, colour, reflecting the depth and nature of disease, and the strength of pathogenic Qi and antipathogenic Qi.

Vitality of the tongue:

- *Moistened tongue*: Rosy with vitality is a favourable sign.

- *Withered tongue*: Dry without lustre is an unfavourable sign.

Colour of the tongue

Colour	Significance	
Pale	Deficiency syndrome	Failure of Yang Qi, which is deficient, to produce enough Blood and push it to the tongue
	Cold syndrome	
	Qi and Blood deficiency	
Red	Fresh red with thorns on the tongue	Excess Heat syndrome
	Fresh red with little coating and cracks on the tongue, or red without coating	Deficient Heat syndrome
Dark red	Exogenous disease, dark red, or with red thorns on the tongue	Febrile disease with Heat entering Blood
	Endogenous disease, dark red, or without coating, or cracks on the tongue	Yin deficiency with Fire flaring
	Moistened with little coating	Blood stasis
Purple	Dark purple and dry	Heat consuming Body Fluid, Qi and Blood stagnation
	Purplish or blue purple and moistened	Cold stagnation with Blood stasis
Blue	Blue in colour	Cold, Blood stasis caused by stagnation of Yang Qi
	Whole tongue is blue	Cold directly affecting Liver and Kidneys, Yang Qi stagnation
	Blue on borders, or thirst but without desire to drink	Blood stasis

Purple-blue tongue can be seen in patients with congenital Heart diseases, and drug or food poisoning

Appearance of the tongue

	Appearance	Significance
Tenderness	Old with rough texture	Excess syndrome
	Tender with fine texture	Deficiency syndrome
Swollen	Bigger, no room in mouth	Accumulation of water and retention of Phlegm
	Pale, tender, moistened coating	Yang deficiency of Spleen and Kidneys, retention of water
	Reddish, bigger, yellow sticky coating	Damp Heat in Spleen and Stomach, Phlegm
Swelling	Occupying the mouth or even unable to withdraw the tongue	Accumulated Heat of Heart and Spleen, excessive Heat in vessels, Qi and Blood going upward, fresh red tongue accompanied with pain Blood stagnated due to poisoning, swollen tongue blue purple in colour without lustre
Thin	Smaller and thinner	Qi and Blood deficiency, failure of blood to fill the tongue
	Smaller, dark red and dry	Yin deficiency with Fire flaring
	Smaller and pale	Qi and Blood deficiency
Spotted, thorny	Red, white or black thorns higher than the tongue surface, granules on the tongue	Evil Heat entering the Blood
	Blue purple or dark purple spots on the tongue, not higher than the tongue surface	Febrile disease, Heat entering Blood, endogenous disease, Blood stasis
Cracked	Irregular streaks or cracks on the tongue	Lack of nourishment because of Yin and Blood deficiency
Glossy	Mirror smooth, without coating	Exhaustion of Stomach-Qi and Yin
Tooth-printed	Swollen tongue with tooth-prints on borders	Spleen deficiency, excessive Damp
Ulcer	Ulcer tongue with pain	Evil Heat of Heart Meridian flaring up, Yin deficiency of Lower Burner
Veins on the under-surface	Normal: light purple, not varicose	
	Purple, thick	Qi stagnation and Blood stasis
	Blue, thin	Cold stagnation with Blood stasis, Yang deficiency causing Qi and Blood circulation not smooth

Movement of the tongue

Stiff tongue

Manifestation	Significance
Stiff tongue with slurred speech	Febrile disease with Heat entering Pericardium, the Mind stored in the Heart getting disturbed, the tongue being without dependence
	High fever exhausting Body Fluid; muscles and tendons lacking nourishment
	Windstroke or its aura
	Liver Wind bringing up Phlegm

Flaccid tongue

Manifestation	Significance	
Soft with difficulty in motion	Qi and Blood deficiency	Muscles and tendons lacking nourishment
	Excessive Heat exhausting Body Fluid	
	Yin deficiency to extreme degree	

Trembling tongue

Manifestation	Significance
Involuntary tremor	Qi and Blood deficiency, collapse of Yang, with Body Fluid exhausted, muscles and tendons lacking nourishment and moisture
	Excessive Heat damaging Body Fluid and producing Wind

Deviated tongue

Manifestation	Significance
Deviated	Meridians and collaterals being attacked by Wind, Wind Phlegm blocking collaterals, Windstroke or its early threatening signs

Wagging tongue

Manifestations	Significance	
Tongue protruded	Epidemic toxin affecting the Heart	Accumulated Heat in Heart and Spleen Meridians, muscles and tendons contracted with wagging
Tongue protruded and withdrawn quickly in wagging motion	Early threatening signs of Wind stirring; maldevelopment of intelligence	

Short tongue

Manifestation	Significance	
Contracted	Cold stagnated in muscles and tendons	Critical condition
	Phlegm retention	
	Excessive Heat exhausting Body Fluid and stirring up Wind	
	Qi and Blood deficiency	

Protruding tongue

Manifestation	Significance
Protruding with difficulty in withdrawing	Excess Heat or Phlegm Fire disturbing the Heart

Paralyzed tongue

Manifestation	Significance
Paralyzed tongue, with numbness and sluggish movement	Failure of Blood to nourish, Blood deficiency causing Liver Wind stirring, Wind bringing up Phlegm

Colour of the tongue-coating

	Manifestations	Significance
White		Exterior syndrome – Taiyang syndrome, Wei stage syndrome
	Pale tongue with white moistened coating	Interior Cold syndrome, Cold Damp
	Powder-like white substance on the tongue, not dry	Interior Heat syndrome seen in pestilence, visceral abscess
	Dry and rough as sandstone	Febrile disease with quick formation of Heat, excessive interior Heat
Yellow	Yellowish indicating mild Heat; dark yellow meaning serious Heat; burnt yellow showing accumulated Heat in the stomach and intestines	Interior syndrome, Heat syndrome
	Changing from white to yellow	Exogenous pathogens going from surface to interior – Yangming syndrome, Qi stage syndrome
	Thin coating in yellowish colour	Wind Heat syndrome of exterior disease, Wind Cold transformed into Heat
	Pale tongue, swollen and tender, with yellow and moistened coating	Failure of Yang deficiency to dissolve Damp
Grey		Interior syndrome – interior Heat syndrome, Cold Damp syndrome
	Grey and dry	Heat excess exhausting the Body Fluid – seen in exterior Heat syndrome, Yin deficiency with Fire flaring
	Grey and moistened	Retention of Phlegm fluid, Cold Damp retention
Black		Interior syndrome – extreme Heat, excessive Cold
	Dry and thorny	Extreme Heat with Body Fluid exhausted
	Moistened	Excess Cold with Yang exhausted
Green		Heat syndrome seen in pestilence, Damp-warm syndrome
Mildew paste-like	Red, black, yellow	Retention of Damp in Stomach and intestines transformed into Heat

Quality of the tongue-coating

	Manifestations	Significance	
Thick-thin	Thin (tongue proper can indistinctly be seen)	Exterior syndrome, mild endogenous disease – antipathogenic Qi not yet damaged	
	Thick (tongue proper cannot be seen)	Pathogens entering interior, retention of Phlegm fluid and food	
Moist-dry	Slippery (over-moistened)	Changes of Body Fluid	Yang deficiency, retention of Phlegm Damp – failure of Yang to dissolve Water
	Dry		Excessive Heat exhausting Body Fluid, exhaustion of Yin fluid, Yang deficiency
	Coarse like sandstone		Excessive Heat exhausting Body Fluid
Sticky-granular	Coarse loose thick granules easily scrubbed off	Excessive Yang	Excessive Yang steaming the turbidity in Stomach – seen in cases with food retention, visceral abscess
	Sticky with fine greasy substance difficult to scrub off	Blockage of Yang Qi	Accumulation of Damp with Yang Qi blocked – seen in cases of Damp, Phlegm, food retention, and Damp Heat
	Yellow sticky		Phlegm Heat, Damp Heat, summer Heat, retention of food, accumulation of Damp Phlegm
	White slippery		Damp, Cold Damp
	White thick sticky coating with a sweet feeling in mouth		Damp Heat in Spleen and Stomach
Uneven distribution	Full distribution	Diffusing of pathogenic Qi, Damp Phlegm in Middle Burner	
	Unevenly distributed — Distributed to tongue tip	Pathogens not deeply entering, Stomach-Qi injured	
	Distributed to tongue root	Exogenous pathogens reduced but still with retention in Stomach	
	Distributed to one side	Pathogens half in exterior and half interior	

Peeled	Peeled completely, a mirror tongue	These states indicate the existence or not of Stomach-Qi and Yin	
	Partially peeled with clear margins		
	Geographic coating with big patches of coating off		
	Peeled unsmooth coating like new granules growing		
Thick to thin	Changing from thick to thin	Antipathogenic Qi restoring	Slow changing is a good sign
Thin to thick	Changing from thin to thick	Pathogenic Qi becoming excessive	
True or false	Rooted coating (firm, not easily scrubbed off)	In the early and middle stage of disease, the rooted coating means that the pathogenic condition is worse. In the late stage of disease, the rooted coating means that the pathogenic condition is getting relieved	
	Without root (not firm, easily scrubbed off)		

Comprehensive observation of the tongue and its coating

Manifestations	Significance
Pale tongue with thin coating	Deficiency Cold of Spleen and Stomach, Water Damp affecting upward
Pale tongue with white dry coating	Heat retention in Spleen and Stomach, Heat injuring Body Fluid
Pale tongue with yellow and cracked coating	Qi deficiency with less Body Fluid
Pale tongue with black and dry coating	Yang deficiency with excessive Cold
Light red tongue without coating	Yin deficiency of Stomach and Kidneys, Qi and Blood deficiency
Light red tongue with white slippery coating	Pathogens half enter the interior, Liver and Gallbladder diseases, Damp changed into dryness damaging Yin, Yin deficiency with prolonged retention of food in Stomach
Light red tongue with white sticky dry coating	Wind Cold affecting, Heat accumulation in Blood, excessive Heat damaging Body Fluid, Damp stagnated in Spleen and Stomach

Manifestations	Significance
Light red root and white tip of tongue with yellow coating	Heat in Upper Burner, invasion of Wind Heat, Wind Cold transformed into Heat entering the interior
Light red tongue with yellow black coating	Phlegm Damp Heat transformed into dryness damaging Yin, Damp Heat in Spleen and Stomach
Red tongue with loose, dirty coating	Deficiency of antipathogenic Qi, Damp Heat not yet completely dissolved
Red tongue with white slippery coating	Interior Heat accompanied with Damp, Yang deficiency with excessive Damp
Red tongue with black slippery coating	Deficiency Cold syndrome
Red borders with black coating in the middle	Internal Cold with external Heat, invasion of summer Heat and eating of Cold raw food, Liver and Stomach Heat with Stomach Cold
Root of tongue is red, coating on the tip of tongue is black	Excessive Heat in the Heart
Red slim tongue with black coating	Body Fluid exhausted with dryness of Blood
Dark red tongue with thin white coating	Constitutionally Yin deficiency with Fire flaring, invasion of Wind Cold; exogenous pathogens not yet completely driven off, Heat entering Blood
Dark red tongue with sticky coating	Body Fluid deficiency, Damp Heat steaming up, Phlegm turbidity
Dark red tongue with yellowish white coating	Pathogens in the Qi stage; Fire in both Qi and Ying stages
Dark red tongue with yellow moistened coating	Heat accompanied with Damp, Heat forcing Water Damp going up
Dark red tongue with yellow sticky coating	Yin deficiency with Heat and with Phlegm fluid
Dark red tongue with yellow granular coating	Heat stagnated in Stomach and intestines
Purple tongue with white sticky coating	Damp Heat in the interior
Blue purple tongue with yellow and slippery coating	Cold stagnated in vessels, food retention in Spleen and Stomach
Purplish tongue with grey coating	Weak constitution, Heat entering Blood
Blue tongue with yellow coating	Cold Damp in the interior

Importance in tongue diagnosis

Special attention should be paid to the following:

1. The vitality and Stomach-Qi of the tongue.

2. Comprehensive observation of the tongue proper and its coating.

3. Dynamic changes of the tongue proper and its coating.

The significance of tongue diagnosis

*   To understand the strength of antipathogenic Qi.

*   To know the location of disease.

*   To diagnose the nature of pathogenic factors.

*   To predict the development of disease.

*   To guide the treating principles.

II. AUSCULTATION AND OLFACTION

1. LISTENING

1.1 Speech

Speaking lustily and coherently: Excess syndrome, Heat syndrome.

Speaking feebly and in low tones: Deficiency syndrome, Cold syndrome.

1.2 Hoarse voice and loss of voice

Hoarse voice or loss of voice with sudden onset: Invasion of exogenous Wind Cold or Wind Heat, Phlegm retention in the Lungs; failure of Lung-Qi in dispersing; Excess syndrome.

Hoarse voice or loss of voice in a prolonged disease: Yin deficiency of Lungs and Kidneys, deficiency Fire burning the Lungs; Body Fluid of the Lungs exhausted; Deficiency syndrome.

Hoarse voice or loss of voice resulted from shouting: Damage of Qi and Yin.

Hoarse voice or loss of voice due to pregnancy: Failure of Kidney-Qi to nourish the throat, caused by the foetus.

1.3 Heavy voice in low tones

Retention of Wind Cold Damp: Failure of Lung-Qi in dispersing, obstruction of nose.

1.4 Talking

Inactive in talking: Deficiency syndrome, Cold syndrome.

Talkative and restless: Excess syndrome, Heat syndrome.

Speaking feebly and biting back: Extreme degree of deficiency of Qi of Middle Burner.

Abnormal changes in speech are pathological manifestations of the Heart-Mind.

Manifestations	Pathogenesis	Significance
Slurred speech	Wind-Phlegm misting the Heart or obstructing the collaterals	Windstroke or its sequellae
Paraphasia	Heart-Qi deficiency, the Mind stored in the Heart lacking nourishment; disturbance of the Mind by Phlegm, Blood stasis, and Qi stagnation	Prolonged disease, old people
Delirium	Heat disturbing the Heart-Mind, Excess syndrome	Heat entering the Pericardium, or the Yangming Fu Excess syndrome
Unconscious, fading, murmuring	Great damage of the Heart-Qi – Deficiency syndrome	Prolonged disease, serious disease
Murmuring to self	Deficiency of the Heart-Qi, the Mind stored in the Heart lacking nourishment – Deficiency syndrome	Epilepsy, depression
Manic	Phlegm Fire disturbing the Heart	Manic mental disorder

1.5 Respiration

	Manifestations		Significance
Dyspnoea (Chuan-asthma)	Hurried breathing with difficulties in lying flat	Excess syndrome manifested with sudden onset, coarse breathing, difficulty in exhaling, protruded eyes, in a sturdy body figure, strong pulse	Excess Heat in the Lungs; retention of Phlegm fluid
		Deficiency syndrome manifested with slow onset, feeble breathing, worse on exertion, difficulty in inhaling, protruded eyes, in a sturdy body figure, strong pulse	Deficiency of Lungs and Kidneys, failure of the Kidneys in receiving Qi
Wheezing (Xiao-asthma)	Hurried breathing with Phlegm gurgling in the throat		Invasion of exogenous Cold stirring up the obstructed Phlegm fluid
Upward movement of Qi	Failure of the Lungs in dispersing Qi going up to block the trachea, causing hurried breathing	Accompanied with fluid vomiting, difficulty being in a lying position	Phlegm fluid retention in chest
		Accompanied with oedema	Invasion of exogenous pathogenic factors causing obstruction of Lung-Qi, so failure of Water distribution
Shortness of Qi	Hurried and short breathing, without Phlegm gurgling in throat	Short breathing, thirst, joint pain, deep pulse	Phlegm fluid retention in chest – Excess syndrome
		Coarse breathing, accompanied with fullness in chest	Retention of Phlegm fluid and Blood stasis – Excess syndrome
		Weak constitution, tiredness	Deficiency of Lung-Qi – Deficiency syndrome
Deficiency of Qi	Feeble short breathing		Deficiency

1.6 Cough

Manifestations		Significance
Characteristics	*Complications*	
In a hurried and stuffy sound		Cold Damp
In a heavy sound	Thin white Phlegm, obstruction of nose	Invasion of Wind Cold
In a low voice	Profuse Phlegm, easy spitting	Cold Damp, or retention of Phlegm fluid
In a clear voice		Dry Heat
Without Phlegm, or with little mucus		Unproductive cough; Fire Heat cough
In a low voice, yellow thick Phlegm, difficulty spitting, dry and sore throat, nasal hot breath		Lung Heat
Whooping cough with haemoptysis		In infants, combination of Wind and hidden Phlegm transformed into Heat blocking in throat
Diphtheria (cough in a dog-barking voice)	Fever, hoarseness, difficulty inhaling	Lung and Kidney Yin deficiency, evil Fire affecting the throat
In a feeble voice, with foam	Shortness of breath	Lung deficiency
Worse at night		Kidney deficiency
Worse in morning		Spleen deficiency, Cold Damp in Large Intestine

1.7 Vomiting

Ou: With sound and vomit.

Dry ou: With sound but no vomit – Stomach-Qi going upward.

Tu: With vomit but no sound.

Manifestations	Significance
Slow vomiting, weak sound, watery vomit	Deficiency Cold
Strong vomiting, strong sound, yellow sticky vomit	Excess Heat
Heat syndrome, jetting vomiting	Heat disturbing the Mind
Eating in morning and vomiting in evening	Stomach Yang deficiency, Spleen and Kidney Yang deficiency
Vomiting and diarrhoea, abdominal pain	Cholera
With desire to drink, vomiting after drinking	Watery vomiting syndrome, retention of fluid in the Stomach
Accompanied with fullness in chest and abdomen, constipation	Turbid Qi of faeces in intestines affecting upward
Accompanied with fullness in chest and pain in hypochondrium	Liver-Qi affecting the Stomach

1.8 Hiccups

These are caused by upward movement of the Stomach-Qi passing the throat, producing a striking sound.

Manifestations	Significance
Sonorous voice, quick onset	Cold or Heat affecting the Stomach
Feeble voice, in a prolonged disease	Stomach-Qi finishing
Frequent strong short hiccups	Excess Heat
Long weak low hiccup	Deficiency Cold
Hiccup rushing upwards in a low voice	Qi deficiency of the Spleen and Stomach, Deficiency Cold syndrome

1.9 Belching

Belching is caused by the Stomach-Qi going upwards. Sighing is a result of Liver-Qi stagnation.

Manifestations		Significance
Characteristics	*Complications*	
Belching with a sour smell	Abdominal distention with indigestion	Qi stagnation in the Stomach
Frequent belching in a sonorous voice followed by relief	Made better or worse by emotions	Liver-Qi affecting the Stomach
Belching in a low voice, without sour smell		Deficiency of the Spleen and Stomach, seen in prolonged disease and old people
Frequent belching aroused by invasion of Cold	Cold pain in epigastric and abdominal region, white tongue-coating	Cold affecting the Stomach

1.10 Sneezing

Sneezing is caused by the rushing upward of Lung-Qi, and is seen in the invasion of Wind Cold syndrome.

1.11 Borborygmus

Borborygmus means the gurgling sound made by the intestines.

Manifestations	Significance
Water wave sound in the epigastric region, standing and walking making the sound reduce	Retention of Phlegm fluid in the Stomach
Made better by warmth and eating, worse by Cold and hunger	Deficiency Cold of the Stomach and Intestines
With a thunder-like sound, fullness in abdomen, watery stools	Wind Cold Damp affecting the Intestines and Stomach
Pain in the abdomen, Cold extremities, vomiting	Excessive Cold
Disappearance of intestinal sound, abdominal distention and pain becoming worse on pressure	Serious Qi stagnation of the Stomach and Intestines

2. SMELLING

A fishy smell or no smell: Deficiency syndrome, Cold syndrome, Cold Damp.

A strongly fishy smell: Excess syndrome, Heat syndrome, Damp Heat.

A stinking and rotten smell: Retention of food.

2.1 Smells of the mouth

Smells of the mouth can help in diagnosis of indigestion, Heat in the Stomach, visceral abscess, and so on.

2.2 Smells of sweat

A smelling of mutton: Retention of Wind Damp Heat in the skin steaming the Body Fluid.

2.3 Smells of Phlegm and nasal discharge

Yellow thick smelly Phlegm: Heat in the Lungs.

Pus-bloody fishy Phlegm: Phlegm Heat accumulated in the Lungs.

Profuse thin Phlegm: Retention of Phlegm fluid in the Lungs.

Profuse smelly turbid nasal discharge: Rhinorrhoea; Lung Heat, Damp Heat in the Gallbladder steaming up.

Running nose: Exterior Wind Cold syndrome.

2.4 Smells of the hospital ward

A smell of urine: Late stage of oedema disease.

A smell of rotting apples: Diabetes.

A smell of blood: Bleeding diseases.

2.5 Smells of vomit

Thin and clear without smell: Stomach Cold.

Turbid and smelly: Stomach Heat.

Sour: Retention of food.

A fishy, bloody smell: Stomach abscess.

2.6 Smells of urine and faeces

Yellow and smelly urine: Damp Heat in the Lower Burner.

Loose and fishy stools: Deficiency Cold of the Spleen and Intestines.

Stinking stools: Accumulated Heat in the intestines.

Stinking stools and flatulence: Retention of food.

2.7 Smells of menstrual flow and leucorrhoea

Menstrual flow smelly: Heat syndrome.

Menstrual flow fishy: Cold syndrome.

Leucorrhoea thin and fishy: Deficiency Cold, Cold Damp.

Leucorrhoea yellow thick and smelly: Damp Heat.

III. INQUIRING

Inquiring means asking the patient or his/her companion about the disease condition in order to understand the onset and development of the disease and the history of previous treatment in order to make a diagnosis and treatment plan.

Inquiring about general conditions: Name, age, gender, marital status, nationality, profession, native place, present address, etc.

Inquiring about life history: Life experience, dietary habits, work and rest, regularity or irregularity of life, etc.

Inquiring about family history and history of past diseases: Family history – health of linear relatives. History of past diseases – health status and main diseases in the past.

Inquiring about onset of disease: The onset, development and whole process of previous treatment of the current disease.

Inquiring about current disease history: This should cover the following: chills and fever, perspiration, defecation and urination, appetite, chest, hearing, thirst, diseases in the past, causes of diseases, menses and leucorrhoea, smallpox and measles in infants.

1. CHILLS AND FEVER

Knowing about these is very necessary for understanding the nature of causative factors, a balance or not of Yin and Yang, and exogenous or endogenous diseases.

1.1 Chills accompanied by fever

Chills: Feeling Cold, without relief with putting on more clothes.

Fever: Body temperature high or normal, feeling hot in the whole body or a certain part.

Chills and fever: Feeling Cold, and accompanied with high body temperature. This is a sign of a struggle between antipathogenic Qi and pathogenic Qi in an exterior syndrome.

Manifestations		Significance
Characteristics	*Complications*	
Severe chills, mild fever	No sweating, aching of the body	Exterior Cold syndrome – invasion of Cold affecting the body surface and injuring Yang
Mild chills, severe fever	Thirst, red face	Exterior Heat syndrome – invasion of Heat causing excessive Yang
Mild fever, aversion to Wind	Spontaneous sweating, superficial pulse that is a bit slow	Exterior Deficiency Cold syndrome – invasion of Wind causing opening of the pores
Chills and fever	Heaviness and pain of the body, irritability, thirst	Summer Heat affecting the body surface
Chills and fever	Heaviness and pain of the head and body, fullness in chest and epigastric region	Damp blocking the body surface
Chills and fever	Dryness in the throat, cough, little Phlegm	Dryness damaging the body surface

Preponderance of antipathogenic Qi and pathogenic Qi

Preponderance of both – severe chills and fever: Strong struggle between the antipathogenic Qi and pathogenic Qi.

Mild pathogenic Qi and declined antipathogenic Qi – mild chills and fever: Not strong struggle between the antipathogenic Qi and pathogenic Qi.

Preponderant pathogenic Qi and declined antipathogenic Qi – severe chills and mild fever: Pathogenic Qi defeating antipathogenic Qi.

1.2 Chills without fever

Chills without fever: Feeling Cold but no fever, seen in Interior Cold syndrome.

Aversion to Cold: Feeling Cold, but relieved by putting on more clothes.

Manifestations	Significance
Excess Cold syndrome – Cold affecting directly, damaging Yang Qi	New disease, a severe Cold pain in epigastrium or other part of the body; deep slow forceful pulse
Deficiency Cold syndrome – deficiency of Yang Qi failing to warm the body	Prolonged disease, weak constitution with aversion to cold; deep slow forceless pulse

1.3 Fever without chills

	Manifestations		Significance
High fever	Persistent high fever (over 39°), red face, thirst, preference for Cold drinks, profuse sweating, surging pulse		Interior Heat syndrome – pathogenic factor entering interior and transformed into Heat, strong struggle between antipathogenic Qi and pathogenic Qi, excessive interior Heat
Tidal fever	Fever occurs, or becomes worse, at a fixed hour of the day just like the waves of the sea	Yangming Heat – tidal fever in the afternoon at 3–5 o'clock, accompanied by abdominal distention and constipation	Yangming Fu Excess syndrome – Heat in Stomach and Large Intestine; Yangming Qi excess in afternoon at 3–5 o'clock plus excess Heat
		Damp Heat – Heat felt in a long palpating; fever becoming worse in the afternoon, accompanied with heaviness of the head and body	Damp Heat in febrile disease – Damp Heat inside the body, so Heat felt in a long palpating. Yang Qi declining in the afternoon, weak in resisting disease, so fever becoming worse in the afternoon

Manifestations		Significance
	Yin deficiency Heat — afternoon or night low fever, feeling like Heat radiating from inside bones, accompanied with flushed cheeks and night sweating	Yin Deficiency syndrome — Yang Qi declines in the afternoon, weak in resisting diseases, the disease is worse, so the fever is worse. At night, defensive Yang enters into the interior, so feels like Heat from inside bones
Low fever	37°–38°	Seen in some endogenous diseases and the late stage of febrile diseases

Classifications according to pathogenesis

Manifestations		Significance
Fever due to Yin deficiency		Same as the Yin deficiency Heat
Fever due to Qi deficiency	Low fever for a long time, worse on exertion, or persistent high fever, accompanied with spontaneous sweating and tiredness	Weakness of Spleen-Qi — failure to disperse clear Yang, which stagnates in the body surface, so causes fever
Infantile summer fever	Long-time fever in summer accompanied with restlessness, thirst, no sweating, and more urine; self-cured when autumn starts	Qi and Yin deficiency of infants failing to adapt to the Heat in summer

1.4 Alternate chills and fever

This is the representative symptom of intermediate syndromes, as is seen in Shaoyang disease and malaria.

Shaoyang Disease

In this there are alternating attacks of chills and fever, accompanied by a bitter taste in the mouth, thirst, a dry throat, a blurring of vision, fullness and stuffiness in the chest and hypochondrium, poor appetite, and a wiry pulse. This is because the exogenous pathogenic factors have stagnated half in the exterior and half in the interior, where the antipathogenic Qi and pathogenic Qi struggle with each other. When the pathogenic Qi is preponderant, chills are present, while when the antipathogenic Qi is preponderant, there is an onset of fever.

Malaria

This causes alternating chills and fever attacks at a fixed time, once a day or every two to three days, accompanied by a severe headache, thirst and profuse sweating. The malaria pathogens stagnate half in the exterior, manifesting as high fever, and half in the interior, manifesting as chills.

2. PERSPIRATION

Sweat is the Body Fluid, steamed by Yang Qi, coming out of the body from the skin pores.

Inquiring about perspiration helps to understand the nature of pathogenic factors, the preponderance of Yin and Yang, and the state of the pores.

2.1 Perspiration in exterior syndrome

Manifestations		Significance
Characteristics	*Complications*	
Exterior syndrome with no sweating	Severe chills, mild fever, neck stiffness, headache, superficial tense pulse	Exterior Cold syndrome – pathogenic Cold is a Yin factor, characterized by contraction. The skin pores are closed, no sweating
Exterior syndrome with sweating	Fever, aversion to Wind, superficial and a pulse that is a bit slow	Exterior Deficient syndrome – pathogenic Wind is a Yang factor, characterized by upward and outward dispersion. The skin pores are open, with Body Fluid coming out
	Severe fever, mild chills, headache, sore throat, superficial rapid pulse	Exterior Heat syndrome – pathogenic Heat is a Yang factor, characterized by upward flaring. The skin pores are open, Body Fluid coming out

2.2 Perspiration in interior syndrome

Manifestations			Significance
Characteristics		*Complications*	
Spontaneous sweating, worse on exertion		Aversion to Cold, tiredness	Yang deficiency – body surface is not strong, Body Fluid comes out. Yang Qi is more exhausted on exertion, sweating becoming worse
Night sweating		Tidal fever, flushed cheeks	Yin deficiency – Yin deficiency transforms into Heat. In sleep, defensive Yang enters the inside, leaving the body surface open. The deficiency Heat forces the Body Fluid out, so there is night sweating. When the patient wakes up, defensive Qi comes from the inside to the body surface, so sweating stops
Profuse sweating	Feeling steaming Heat with continuous sweating	Red face, thirst with preference for Cold drinks, surging pulse	Exogenous pathogenic factor enters the inside, or Wind Heat transmits to the interior. The internal Heat is strong, steaming the Body Fluid out
	Profuse Cold sweat like pearls	Pale complexion, Cold hands and feet, thready fading pulse	Collapse of Yang – when Yang Qi collapses, Body Fluid is out of control, coming out
Perspiration after shivering			In a febrile disease, the antipathogenic Qi and pathogenic Qi struggle fiercely, serving as a turning point of disease
		Chilly perspiration is a turning point of the disease becoming better or worse	After sweating, fever is stopped and pulse becomes normal, indicating that the pathogen is removed and antipathogenic Qi is restored
			After sweating, fever is not stopped and pulse becomes rapid, indicating that the pathogen has become stronger and antipathogenic Qi has declined. The pathological condition changes to worse

2.3 Perspiration in a local part

Manifestations		Significance
Characteristics	*Complications*	
Head and neck sweating		Excessive Heat in Upper Burner, Damp Heat in Middle Burner, deficiency Yang floating up
Heat sweating	Heaviness of head and body, feverishness, chest fullness, yellow, sticky tongue-coating	Damp Heat in febrile disease – Damp Heat of Middle Burner steams upward to the facial region
Half of body sweating		The meridians and collaterals of that half of the body are obstructed, consequently Qi and Blood circulation are blocked, seen in Windstroke, Wei syndrome and paraplegic patients
Palm and sole sweating		Yang Qi stagnated inside, Damp Heat in Middle Burner, Yin deficiency with internal Heat
Chest sweating		Deficiency of Heart and Spleen, disharmony between Heart and Kidneys

3. THE HEAD AND BODY

3.1 Headache

Quick onset, short course, severe continuous headache: Exogenous headache, Excess syndrome.

Slow onset, long course, dull non-continuous headache: Endogenous headache, Deficiency syndrome.

Headache on the lateral side: Shaoyang headache.

Headache in the occipital region and nape: Taiyang headache.

Headache on the top: Jueyin headache.

Headache radiating to teeth: Shaoyin headache.

Manifestations	Significance
Headache with aversion to heat, red face and eyes	Exogenous headache – Wind Heat disturbing the head
Headache with the nape involved and worsened by exposure to Wind	Exogenous headache – Wind Cold blocking the Taiyang Meridian
A heavy sensation in the head as though it had been wrapped in a piece of cloth; heaviness of the body as though it were carrying a heavy load	Exogenous headache – Wind Damp blocking Yang Qi, causing a failure of clear Yang ascending
A dull headache aggravated by overstrain	Qi deficiency headache – Qi deficiency of Middle Burner, failure of clear Yang in ascending
Headache, dizziness, pale complexion	Blood deficiency headache – Blood deficiency causes a failure to nourish the head
Headache, dizziness, unclear-minded	Spleen deficiency causes a failure of clear Yang in ascending
Hollow-like headache, soreness in lumbus and knees	Kidney deficiency headache – deficiency of Kidney Essence, Sea of Marrow not well filled up

3.2 Dizziness

Manifestations		Significance
Characteristics	*Complications*	
Dizziness with a distending feeling in head	Red face, tinnitus, bitter taste in mouth, dry throat	Liver Yang hyperactivity – the hyperactive Yang disturbing the head, hyperactivity of Yang causing the Wind
Dizziness with a heavy feeling in head	Fullness in chest, nausea, sputum in throat	Phlegm Damp retention causing a failure of clear Yang ascending
Dizziness with blurred vision, worse by overstrain and sudden standing-up	Pale complexion, pale tongue, palpitation, insomnia	Qi and Blood deficiency giving poor nourishment to the brain
Dizziness, tinnitus	Seminal emission, forgetfulness, soreness in the lumbus and knees	Deficiency of Kidney Essence, Sea of Marrow not well filled up, poor nourishment to the brain

3.3 Body

	Manifestations	Significance
Aching of body	Aching all over the body	Invasion of Wind Cold Damp – meridians and collaterals are blocked, Qi and Blood circulation is stagnated
	Yang toxin (red face with spots, body aches as if hit by stick)	Invasion of summer Heat and Damp – Qi and Blood circulation is stagnated by pestilence
	Aching all over the body in a prolonged disease	Blood deficiency, disharmony between Qi and Blood
Heaviness of body	Heavy sensation in the head and body, fullness in epigastrium, poor appetite, loose stools	Invasion of Damp – Damp blocking the meridians and collaterals
	Heavy sensation in the body, somnolence, inactive in talking, listlessness	Spleen-Qi deficiency – failure of Spleen in transportation and transformation causing poor nourishment of muscles
Pain of limbs	Bi syndrome (pain of joints of limbs)	Invasion of Wind Cold Damp
	Wandering Bi (migrating pain of joints)	Invasion of Wind – pathogenic Wind is characterized by moving, thus the pain is wandering
	Painful Bi (severe pain of joints)	Invasion of Cold – pathogenic Cold is characterized by contraction, thus Qi and Blood are stagnated.
	Fixed Bi (fixed pain of joints)	Invasion of Damp – pathogenic Damp is characterized by viscosity and stagnation, thus Qi and Blood are stagnated
	Heat Bi (redness, swelling and pain of joints)	Wind Damp transforming into Heat
Pain of lumbus	Soreness and weakness in the lumbar region	Kidney deficiency – Kidney Essence is deficient, bone is not well filled up with marrow, lumbus is lacking nourishment
	Cold pain and heaviness in the lumbus, worse on rainy days	Cold Damp – invasion of Cold Damp to the lumbus, blocking the meridians and collaterals and stagnating Qi and Blood
	Stabbing pain in the lumbus, fixed in place, worse on pressure, motor impairment	Blood stasis – Blood stasis blocking the meridians and collaterals and stagnating Qi and Blood

3.4 Chest, hypochondrium, epigastrium, abdomen

Chest

Manifestations	Significance
Chest Bi (choking pain in the chest referring to the shoulder and back)	Obstruction of Yang Qi in chest with retention of Phlegm; Qi deficiency with Blood stasis, stagnation of Qi and Blood in the Heart
Real Heart pain (severe pain in the chest referring to the back, grey complexion, cyanosis of hands and feet)	Heart vessels are obstructed suddenly
Chest pain, high fever, red face, abrupt breathing, nares flaring	Excess Heat syndrome of the Lungs
Chest pain, tidal fever, night sweating, cough with bloody sputum	Yin Deficiency syndrome of the Lungs
Fullness in chest, cough, asthmatic breathing, profuse white sputum	Phlegm Damp affecting the Lungs
Pulmonary abscess (chest pain, fever, cough with purulent sputum)	Heat accumulated in the Lungs, stagnation of Qi and Blood, flesh going bad into purulence
Distending and migrating pain in the chest, sighing, hot temper	Qi stagnation, obstruction of Qi in the chest
Fixed stabbing pain in chest	Blood stasis blocking the meridians and collaterals of the chest
Fullness in chest, no pain, Cold sensation in chest, cough with sputum froth, slow pulse	A cord-like mass and pain in the hypochondrium caused by Cold
Fullness in chest, no pain, irritability, thirst, rapid pulse	Glomus-like mass caused by Heat
Fullness in chest, no pain, listlessness, unsmooth breathing, weak pulse, sighing	Stuffy sensation caused by exhaustion of Yin, Yang, and Blood
Fullness in chest, no pain, profuse sputum, rolling pulse	Accumulation of Phlegm in hypochondrium

Hypochondrium

Manifestations	Significance
Distending pain, sighing, hot temper	Liver-Qi stagnation, emotional depression
Burning pain, redness of face and eyes	Liver Fire burning the collaterals of the hypochondrium
Distending pain, jaundice	Damp Heat of Liver and Gallbladder
Fixed stabbing pain	Blood stasis blocking the meridians and collaterals
Fluid retention in the hypochondrium manifested as pain and fullness of costal region, which is made worse by cough	Fluid retention in the hypochondrium
Fullness and pain, alternate chills and fever	Shaoyang syndrome

Epigastrium

Manifestations	Significance
Severe Cold pain, made better by warmth	Invasion of Stomach by Cold – Cold injuring the Stomach Yang, the contraction of Stomach causing the pain
Burning pain, voracious eating, bad smell from mouth, constipation	Stomach Fire excess
Distending pain, belching, made worse by emotional factors	Qi stagnation of the Stomach
Fixed stabbing pain	Blood stasis blocking the collaterals of the Stomach
Dull pain, made better by warmth and pressure, vomiting with clear fluid	Yang deficiency produces Cold, which causes the hypofunction of the Stomach
Burning pain, hunger but with no desire to eat, red tongue, little coating	Yin deficiency of the Stomach – deficiency of Yin and Body Fluid, deficiency Fire disturbing the Stomach

Abdomen

Manifestations	Significance
Acute, severe distending pain, made worse by pressure and food-intake	Excess syndrome
Dull pain, better by pressure and food-intake	Deficiency syndrome
A pain getting better by warmth	Cold syndrome
A pain getting better by Cold	Heat syndrome
Dull pain, better by warmth and pressure, loose stools	Deficiency Cold of Spleen and Stomach, disturbance of transportation and transformation
Distending pain in the lower abdomen, dysuria	Retention of urine due to dysfunctions of Bladder Qi activities
Cold pain in the lower abdomen, referring to the perineum	Cold stagnated in the Liver Meridian causing the contraction
A movable mass and pain around the umbilicus	Worm accumulation

4. THE EARS AND EYES

Consideration of manifestations in the ears and eyes enables diagnosis of local diseases and diseases of the Liver, Gallbladder, and Kidneys.

	Manifestations	**Significance**
Tinnitus	Sudden onset, loud sound, made worse by pressure	Excess syndrome – Fire of Liver, Gallbladder and Triple Burner moving upward to the ear
	Slow onset, cicada-singing-like sound, made better or stopped by pressure	Deficiency syndrome – Damp of Spleen causing failure of clear Yang ascending; deficiency of Kidney Essence giving poor nourishment to the ears
Deafness	Sudden onset	Liver and Gallbladder Fire; traumatic injury; drug poisoning
	Prolonged	Deficiency of Kidney Essence
Hearing impairment	Not hearing clearly	Pathogenic Wind; Heat in the Liver Meridian, deficiency of Kidney Essence
Pain of eyes	Severe pain, headache, nausea, vomiting, dilated pupils like cloudy patches in green or yellow colour	Bluish glaucoma
Dizziness	Accompanied with distention in the head, red face, tinnitus, soreness in lumbus and knees	Kidney Yin deficiency, Liver Yang hyperactivity
	Accompanied by fullness in the chest, tiredness, numbness of extremities, nausea, sticky tongue-coating	Retention of Phlegm Damp, failure of clear Yang ascending
Blurred vision	Dry sensation in eyes, blurring of vision	Qi deficiency, Liver Blood deficiency, Kidney Essence deficiency, poor nourishment of eyes
Night blindness		Deficiency of Liver and Kidney, deficiency of Essence and Blood

5. APPETITE, THIRST AND TASTE

Inquiring about appetite, thirst and taste helps to understand the sufficiency-or-not and distribution of Body Fluid, the function of the Spleen and the Stomach and the sufficiency-or-not of food Essence.

5.1 Thirst and drinking

Inquiring about thirst and drinking helps to understand the sufficiency-or-not and distribution of Body Fluid. Thirst but not drinking much indicates distribution disturbance of Body Fluid.

Manifestations			Significance
Characteristics	*Complications*		
No thirst			No damage of Body Fluid
Thirst and drinking a lot			Serious damage of Body Fluid
Thirst and drinking a lot	Preference for Cold drinks	High fever, irritability, sweating, surging pulse	Excess Heat syndrome – excessive internal Heat, serious damage of Body Fluid
	Drinking a lot, profuse urine	Eating a lot, emaciation	Diabetes – Kidney Yin deficiency, Kidney Yang hyperactivity, more opening and less closing of Bladder
	After sweating, vomiting and diarrhoea		Damage of Body Fluid
Thirst but without drinking a lot			Yin deficiency, Damp Heat, Phlegm, Blood stasis
Dry mouth, without desire to drink	Tidal fever, night sweating, flushed cheeks		Yin Deficiency syndrome – insufficiency of Body Fluid with failure to moisten the mouth, so dry mouth; without exhaustion of Body Fluid caused by excess Heat, so no desire to drink
Thirst but not drinking a lot	Heaviness of the head and body-Heat felt in a long palpating, fullness in epigastrium, sticky tongue-coating		Damp Heat syndrome – disturbance of Body Fluid distributing to the mouth, so thirst; Damp retention causing not drinking a lot

| Preferring hot drinks but not drinking a lot, or vomiting immediately after drinking | Dizziness, blurred vision, watery sound in Stomach and Intestines | Retention of Phlegm – Phlegm is a Yin pathogenic factor, damaging Yang, thus Body Fluid cannot be steamed upward to moisten the mouth, so thirst with preference of hot drinks. Retention of Phlegm fluid causes the failure of Stomach-Qi in descending, so vomiting occurs immediately after drinking. This is a disturbance of distribution of Body Fluid |
| Dry mouth with preference for holding water in throat but not drinking | Dark purple tongue with spots of Blood stasis, hesitant pulse | Blood stasis – disturbance of distribution of Body Fluid due to Blood stasis causing no moisture to the mouth |

5.2 Appetite and amount of food eaten

Inquiring about appetite and amount of food eaten helps in understanding the functioning of the Spleen and Stomach.

Reduced appetite

Manifestations		Significance
Characteristics	*Complications*	
Poor appetite	Emaciation, tiredness, abdominal distention, loose stools, pale tongue, weak pulse	Qi deficiency of Spleen and Stomach – hypofunction of transportation and transformation, seen in prolonged Deficiency syndrome
Fullness in epigastrium, poor appetite	Heaviness of head and body, loose stools, sticky tongue-coating	Damp affecting the Spleen – failure of Spleen in transportation and transformation
Poor appetite with dislike of oil-cooked food	Jaundice, hypochondria pain, fever	Damp Heat of Liver and Gallbladder – accumulation of Damp Heat, failure of Liver in keeping free flow of Qi, failure of Spleen in transportation and transformation
Anorexia	Belching, distending pain in epigastrium, thick tongue-coating	Retention of food – voracious eating damaging the Spleen and Stomach, causing a disorder in transportation and transformation
Women of child-bearing age with vomiting and dislike of eating, rolling pulse		Vomiting during pregnancy is a normal physiological phenomenon

Eating a lot but still hungry

Manifestations		Significance
Characteristics	*Complications*	
Excessive appetite, eating a lot, but skinny		Heat accumulates in the Stomach, making the food Essence exhausted
Overeating but hungry	Thirst, irritability, red tongue, yellow coating, bad smell from mouth, constipation	Stomach Fire excess – hyperactivity of metabolism
	Loose stools	Strong Stomach but weak Spleen – hyperfunction of Stomach in receiving food but hypofunction of Spleen in transportation and transformation

Hungry but no desire to eat

Manifestations		Significance
Characteristics	*Complications*	
Feel hungry but no desire to eat or eat very little	Burning sensation in Stomach, red tongue, little coating, thready and rapid pulse	Stomach Yin insufficiency, deficiency Fire disturbing

Special preferences for types of food

Manifestations	Significance
Preference for rich food	Producing Phlegm Damp
Preference for Cold and raw food	Damaging Spleen and Stomach
Preference for spicy food	Inducing dryness and Heat
Craving for raw rice or earth	Infantile parasitic diseases

5.3 Taste

Manifestations	Significance
Food seeming tasteless	Qi deficiency of Spleen and Stomach – hypofunction of transportation and transformation, so poor appetite
Sweet taste or sticky feeling in mouth	Damp Heat of Spleen and Stomach – sweet entering Spleen, accumulation of Damp Heat in Spleen and Stomach, turbid Qi going upward to the mouth
Sour taste in mouth	Accumulated Heat of Liver and Stomach – sour entering Liver, Liver Heat going upward to the mouth
Sour stale taste in mouth	Retention of food – overeating damaging Spleen and Stomach, turbid Qi of retained food going upward to the mouth
Bitter taste in mouth	Heat syndrome; Gallbladder Heat going upward
Salty taste in mouth	Kidney deficiency; Cold syndrome – Water Cold in Kidney disease affecting upward
Hypoesthesia due to numbness	Liver Yang transforming into Wind; overdose of drugs
Pain in the mouth	Accumulation of Heat in Spleen and Stomach; Heart Fire flaring up; Yin deficiency causing Fire flaring

6. SLEEP

Inquiring about sleep helps in diagnosing the functional conditions of Qi and Blood and the Zang Fu organs.

	Manifestations		Significance
	Characteristics	*Complications*	
Insomnia	Difficulty in falling asleep	Irritability, dream-disturbed sleep, tidal fever, night sweating, soreness and weakness in lumbus and knees	Disharmony between Heart and Kidneys – Kidney Yin deficiency, Heart Fire flaring, the Mind stored in the Heart getting disturbed
	Easily awoken	Palpitations, poor appetite, tiredness, pale tongue, weak pulse	Deficiency of both Heart and Spleen – failure of Spleen in transportation and transformation to produce enough Qi and Blood causing Heart Blood deficiency, the Mind stored in the Heart lacking nourishment
	Light sleep	Dizziness, fullness in chest, timidity, irritability, bitter taste in mouth, nausea	Gallbladder stagnation with attacking of Phlegm – restlessness of Gallbladder-Qi, Mind restlessness
	Difficulty in sleeping for the whole night	Fullness in epigastrium, belching, abdominal distention, thick sticky tongue-coating	Food retention – improper eating damaging Spleen and Stomach, failure of Stomach-Qi to go downward, turbid Qi disturbing upward, the Mind stored in the Heart getting disturbed 'Stomach discomfort causes poor sleep'
Somnolence	Sleepiness, easy to fall asleep	Dizziness, heaviness in the head and body, fullness in epigastrium, sticky tongue-coating, thready soft pulse	Affecting of Spleen by Phlegm Damp – failure of clear Yang in ascending, poor nourishment to the head
	Sleepiness, easy to fall asleep after meals	Weak constitution, poor appetite, tiredness	Spleen-Qi deficiency – failure of clear Yang in ascending, poor nourishment to the head
	Extreme tiredness, clear consciousness, easy to fall asleep	Cold extremities, feeble pulse	Decline of Heart and Kidney Yang – Yin Cold excess, hypofunction of Zang Fu organs
	Lethargy with delirium	Fever becoming worse at night, macule, dark red tongue, rapid pulse	Heat entering Ying Blood – pathogen entering Pericardium, misting the Mind, and leading to unconsciousness

7. STOOLS AND URINE

Inquiring about stools and urine helps in diagnosing the functioning of the Lungs, Spleen, Kidney, Small and Large Intestines and Bladder and the nature of any diseases present.

7.1 Stools

Constipation: Deficiency of Body Fluid in Large Intestine, which fails to carry out transportation of faeces.

Diarrhoea: Failure of Spleen in transportation and transformation, Water blocking in Large Intestine, which fails to carry out normal transportation.

Abnormal frequency of defecation

	Manifestations	Significance
Constipation	High fever, distending pain in abdomen, red tongue with yellow dry coating	Excess Heat syndrome – Heat exhausting the Body Fluid, dryness of Large Intestine
	Pale complexion, preference for hot drinks, deep and slow pulse	Cold constipation – accumulation of Yin Cold, obstruction of Qi of intestines
	Dry stools, red tongue with little coating, thready rapid pulse	Yin deficiency – deficiency of Body Fluid, intestines not well moistened
	Prolonged disease, old age, after delivery	Qi deficiency – no power to push faeces, Body Fluid deficiency giving no moisture to intestines
Diarrhoea	Poor appetite, abdominal distention with a dull pain, loose stools	Spleen deficiency – failure of Spleen in transportation and transformation, failure of Small Intestine in separating the turbid from the clear, Water stagnating in intestines
	Diarrhoea at dawn, weakness and soreness in the lumbus and knees	Kidney Yang deficiency – failure of Kidney Yang to warm Spleen Yang, causing the failure of Spleen in transportation and transformation, Yang Qi in weakness and Yin Qi in preponderance at dawn, and so abdominal pain and diarrhoea
	Fullness in epigastrium, belching, abdominal pain, diarrhoea, relief of abdominal pain after diarrhoea	Overeating – damage of Spleen and Stomach, hyperfunction of Large Intestine in transmission. Turbidity is discharged after diarrhoea, so relief of abdominal pain
	Emotional depression, abdominal pain, diarrhoea, relief of abdominal pain after diarrhoea	Liver Wood stagnation overacting on Spleen Earth

Abnormal quality of stools

Manifestations		Significance
With undigested food in stools		Spleen deficiency, Kidney deficiency
Loose stools, dry stools	Sometimes dry, sometimes loose	Liver stagnation overacting on Spleen
	First dry then loose	Spleen deficiency
Bloody stools	Black	Far Blood
	Fresh red	Near Blood
	Pus in Blood	Dysentery

Abnormal feelings on defecation

Manifestations	Significance
Burning sensation of anus	Damp Heat of Large Intestine
Unsmooth defecation	Liver stagnation overacting on Spleen, Qi stagnation in Intestines
Loose stools with bad smell, lumpy discharge	Damp Heat accumulated in Large Intestine, Qi stagnation of Large Intestine
Tenesmus	Retention of Damp Heat, Qi stagnation of Large Intestine
Uncontrolled stools in prolonged diarrhoea	Spleen and Kidney Yang deficiency, failure of anus in controlling
Bearing-down sensation in anus, even prolapse of rectum	Spleen deficiency with Qi of Middle Burner sinking

7.2 URINE

Inquiring about urine helps in diagnosing the condition of Body Fluid and the functioning of the Lungs, Spleen, and Kidneys.

Abnormal quantity of urine

	Manifestatons	Significance
Increased	Increased volume of clear urine, aversion to cold, preference for warmth	Deficiency Cold syndrome – Body Fluid not damaged because of lack of sweating, Water descending
	Thirst, drinking a lot, urinating a lot, loss of weight	Diabetes – Kidney Yin deficiency, opening more closing less
Decreased	Yellow scanty urine	Excess Heat syndrome; Body Fluid getting damaged after sweating, vomiting and diarrhoea – formation of source of urine getting decreased
	Scanty urine, oedema	Oedema – abnormal functions of Lung, Spleen and Kidney, disorder of Qi activities, Water Damp retention

Abnormal frequency of urination

Manifestations		Significance
Frequent	Stranguria (scanty urine but painful and dripping urination)	Damp Heat accumulation in Lower Burner, disorder of Qi activities of Bladder
	Clear urine, incontinence of urine	Weakness of Kidney-Qi, failure of Bladder in controlling urine
	Increased nocturnal urination, clear urine in increased volume	Deficiency of Kidney Yang, disorder of opening and closing, failure of Bladder in controlling urine, late stage of Kidney diseases
Retention of urine		Damp Heat accumulation, obstruction by Blood stasis or stone, old people with Qi deficiency, Kidney Yang deficiency, disorder of Qi activities of Bladder

Abnormal feeling when urinating

Manifestations	Significance
Stranguria (burning painful and dripping urination)	Damp Heat accumulation in Bladder, disorder of Qi activities of bladder
Dripping urination	Weakness of Kidney-Qi in the aged
Urinary incontinence	Weakness of Kidney-Qi, failure of Bladder in controlling urine
Enuresis	Deficiency of Kidney-Qi, asthenia of Bladder

8. MENSES AND LEUCORRHOEA

Irregular menstruation

	Manifestations	Significance
8–9 days early	Dark red, thick, large quantity	Blood Heat – Blood accelerated
	Light red, thin, large quantity	Qi deficiency – failure of Qi to control Blood
8–9 days late	Light red, thin, small quantity	Blood deficiency – failure of uterus to be fully filled
	Dark purple, with clots, small quantity	Cold stagnation – Blood stagnated due to invasion of Cold, failing to come on time
More than 8–9 days early or late	Purple red, with clots, small quantity, distending pain in breasts	Qi stagnation – emotional depression, failure of Liver in keeping free flow of Qi, disorder of Qi circulation
	Light red, thin, small or large quantity	Deficiency of Spleen and Kidneys, Chong-Ren disorders, failure of Spleen in controlling Blood, Kidney deficiency, Blood deficiency

Dysmenorrhoea	Distending pain occurring in lower abdomen before menstruation and relieved after flow	Excess syndrome – Qi stagnation with Blood stasis, obstruction causing the pain
	Dull pain in lower abdomen after menstruation, soreness in lumbus	Deficiency syndrome – Qi and Blood deficiency, Kidney deficiency, uterus lacking nourishment
Amenorrhoea (for more than 3 months)		Blood stasis; Liver-Qi stagnation, overexertion asthenia
Metrorrhagia and metrostaxis	Dark red, with clots	Heat syndrome
	Light red, without clots	Damage of Chong-Ren, sinking of Qi of Middle Burner, failure of Spleen in controlling Blood

Leucorrhoea

Manifestations	Significance
In white colour, large quantity, thin, no smell	Cold Damp, failure of Spleen in transportation and transformation, downward pouring of Cold Damp
In yellow colour, large quantity, thick, bad smell	Damp Heat pouring downward
In red or red white colour, thick, slightly bad smell	Transformation of Liver stagnation into Heat damaging uterine collaterals

Pregnancy

Manifestations		Significance
Pregnant vomit	Tiredness, can't taste, abdominal distention	Stomach-Qi deficiency, Qi of Chong-Thoroughfare Vessel rushing upward, Stomach-Qi ascending
	Hot temper, acid vomit	Transformation of Liver stagnation into Fire attacking the Stomach
	Fullness in epigastrium, poor appetite, vomiting fluid	Phlegm fluid going upward, Stomach-Qi going up
Threatened abortion		Abortion, threatened abortion

Symptoms after delivery

	Manifestations	Significance
Lochiorrhoea (for more than 20 days)	Large quantity, pale colour, thin quality, sallow complexion, tiredness	Sinking of Qi
	Large quantity, dark red, thick quality, red face, thirst, constipation, yellow urine	Blood accelerated by Heat
	Dark red with clots, stabbing pain in lower abdominal which is made worse by pressure, dark tongue with spots of Blood stasis	Blood stasis
Fever	Aversion to Cold, headache and aching of the body	Exterior syndrome
	High fever, irritability, thirst with preference for Cold drinks, constipation, dark yellow urine	Excess Fire
	Low fever, dull pain in abdomen, dizziness, pale complexion, dry stools	Blood deficiency transformed into dryness producing Heat

9. INFANTS

Physiological characteristics: Delicate Zang Fu organs, vigorous vitality, rapid growth.

Pathological characteristics: Quick onset of diseases, rapid changes in pathological condition, easy excess and easy deficiency.

9.1 Before and after birth

Newborn (after birth to one month): The mother's nutrition and health before and after the delivery, including diseases, medication, difficulty of labour, premature delivery and so on should be inquired about.

Infants (one month to 3 years old): The feeding method, and progress in sitting, crawling, standing and walking, teeth occurrence, and ability to talk should be inquired about.

9.2 History

History of vaccination, infectious diseases, and contact with infectious diseases should be inquired about.

9.3 Cause of disease

The cause of diseases, including the six exogenous pathogenic factors, unbalanced diet, being frightened and so on, should be inquired about.

IV. PALPATION

FORMATION OF THE PULSE

The cardiac impulse is the power of pulse formation: The Heart pushes Blood into the blood vessels to form the pulse.

Qi and Blood circulation is the basis of pulse formation: The Blood moves into the Blood vessel by means of the Zong-pectoral Qi.

The coordination of the five Zang organs is the premise of the normal pulse: The convergence of vessels in the Lungs is for gas exchange. The Spleen and Stomach produce Blood and the Spleen controls Blood. The Liver stores Blood, regulates the circulation volume of Blood, and maintains the free flow of Qi. The Kidneys store Essence which produces Qi, being the motivating power for the functional activities of the Zang Fu organs. The Essence produces Blood.

1. FEELING THE PULSE

1.1 The significance of feeling the pulse

1. To diagnose the location and nature of disease and the relative strength of antipathogenic Qi and pathogenic Qi.

2. To make a prognosis.

1.2 The location for feeling the pulse

Three portions and nine pulse-takings

The pulse is taken on three parts of the body – the head, the upper limbs and the lower limbs – in each of which there are the Heaven, Earth and Human levels.

Three parts of the body

These were first identified in *Treatise on Febrile and Miscellaneous Diseases* by Zhang Zhongjing: Renying (ST 9), Cunkou (ulnar artery at Shenmen (HT 7)) and Fuyang (BL 59).

The Cunkou pulse

This is found in the area on the wrist over the radial artery.

a. Theoretical evidence for Cunkou pulse diagnosis: The origin of the pulse is from the Stomach, running to the Spleen, to the Zang Fu organs, and to the Lungs, in the process of which the influence of Zang Fu diseases is reflected on the radial artery at the wrist.

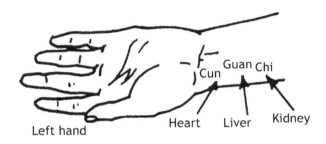

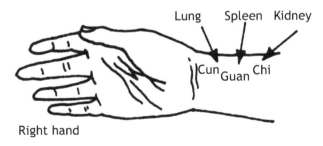

Figure 2.2: Cunkou pulse diagnosis

b. Cunkou pulse

Pulse	Left hand	Right hand
Cun	Heart	Lungs
Guan	Liver and Gallbladder	Spleen and Stomach
Chi	Kidneys	Kidneys

c. Method of feeling the pulse:

- *Time*: Better in the morning. The patient should take a short rest before pulse-taking. The clinic should be kept quiet.

- *Position*: The patient is in a sitting or supine position with his hand stretched out, at the same level as the Heart, palm facing upward. A pulse-pillow should be put under the wrist joint.

- *Doctor's fingers*: Put the middle finger on Guan, index finger on Cun, and ring finger on Chi, and feel the pulse with the finger-pad. The fingers should be slightly flexed, presenting the shape of an arch, naturally close to each other.

- *Procedure*: The three fingers press the three parts together; each finger presses the same part each time.

- *Superficial pressing and deep pressing*: Cun, Guan and Chi are each pressed lightly (superficial palpation), moderately, and heavily (deep palpation), so there are three portions and nine pulse-takings.

- *One breath*: Exhale once and inhale once.

- *Fifty beats*: Each time feeling the pulse should be at least as long a time as 50 beats on each side, 3–5 minutes.

1.3 Pulse essentials
1.3.1 Pulse essentials to note

- Depth (superficial or deep).

- Speed (rapid or slow) and rhythm.

- Shape (thick or thready, soft or hard, long or short).

- Fluency (smooth or hesitant).

- Strength (forceful or weak).

1.3.2 Normal pulse

A normal pulse, with Wei (Stomach), Shen (vitality), and Gen (root), is smooth, even, and forceful, with the frequency of four beats per breath (72–80 beats per minute). However, the pulse may vary according to age, sex, body constitution, emotional state, tiredness and climatic changes.

		Manifestations	Significance
Even	*Wei* (Stomach)	Not superficial not deep, not rapid not slow, even and regular	To diagnose the functions of Spleen and Stomach, conditions of Qi and Blood, and turning of disease
	Shen (Vitality)	Even and forceful in regular rhythm	To diagnose the condition of Heart-Qi and vitality of the patient
Root		Chi pulse is forceful in heavy palpation	To diagnose the status of Kidney Essence and Kidney-Qi

The pulse may vary according to age, sex, body constitution, emotional state, and climatic changes.

- *Oblique running pulse (Xie Fei Mai)*: A pulse that occurs from Chi to the dorsum of the hand.

- *Wrist dorsum radial pulse (Fan Guan Mai)*: A pulse that occurs on the dorsum of Cunkou.

Abnormal pulse readings

A. Fu (superficial), San (scattered), Kou (hollow), Ge (tympanic)

- *Superficial pulse (Fu Mai)*: This can be easily felt with a gentle touch. Its strength is slightly reduced but is not hollow on a little heavy pressing. It indicates exterior and Deficiency syndromes. Because the pathogenic factor locates at the superficial part of the body and the defensive Qi resists the pathogenic factor in the superficial part of the body, in a prolonged disease, if the pulse is superficial, it is always forceless.

- *Scattered pulse (San Mai)*: This is diffusing and feeble with fewer beats on light touch and faint on hard pressing. It indicates exhaustion of Yuan-primary Qi and failure of functions of the Zang Fu organs.

- *Hollow pulse (Kou Mai)*: This feels floating, large, soft, and hollow, like a scallion stalk. It indicates severe loss of blood and the collapse of Yin. Because the volume of blood is suddenly reduced when there is a severe loss of blood, the Body Fluid is greatly damaged and Yin collapses with the Blood loss, so Yang loses its dependence, floating outside.

- *Tympanic pulse (Ge Mai)*: This feels extremely taut and hollow, giving a feeling like touching the surface of a drum. It indicates severe loss of blood, spermatorrhoea, abortion and metrostaxis. Because the antipathogenic Qi is very weak and Essence and Blood are not stored well, the Qi loses its dependence, floating outside.

Comparison

	Manifestations		Significance	
Fu Mai (Superficial)	Easily felt with gentle touch, slightly reduced but not hollow on a little heavy pressure	Superficial but forceful	Exterior syndromes	Exterior Excess syndrome
				Exterior Deficiency syndrome
	Superficial and forceless in a prolonged disease		Yin fails to control Yang, which is floating outside	
San Mai (Scattered)	Diffusing and feeble, with fewer beats on light touch and faint on hard pressing		Exhaustion of Yuan-primary Qi and failure of functions of Zang Fu organs	
Kou Mai (Hollow)	Feels floating, large, soft, and hollow, like a scallion stalk		Severe loss of blood and collapse of Yin	
Ge Mai (Tympanic)	Taut and hollow, giving the feeling of touching the surface of a drum		Severe loss of blood, spermatorrhoea, abortion and metrostaxis	

The physiological superficial pulse may be seen in people who are skinny. The superficial pulse may also be seen in summer and autumn seasons because Yang Qi floats outside.

B. Chen (deep), Fu (hidden), Lao (firm)

- *Deep pulse (Chen Mai)*: This is felt only on pressing hard. It indicates interior syndromes. Because the pathogenic Qi is stagnated inside and Qi and Blood are disturbed, the pulse is deep and forceful, while the antipathogenic Qi is weak and Yang Qi fails to activate strongly, so the pulse is forceless.

- *Hidden pulse (Fu Mai)*: This is felt only on pressing hard to the bone, and is located even deeper than the deep pulse. It indicates syncope, severe pains, and retention of the pathogenic factor in the interior of the body. Because the pathogenic Qi is stagnated inside the body, the vessels are obstructed.

- *Firm pulse (Lao Mai)*: This feels firm, forceful, large, taut and long on pressing hard. It indicates the accumulation of Yin Cold and occurrence of masses because of the firm stagnation of pathogenic Qi inside the body.

Comparison

	Manifestations		Significance	
Chen Mai (Deep)	Felt only on pressing hard	Deep and forceful	Interior syndromes	Interior Excess syndrome
		Deep and forceless		Interior Deficiency syndrome
Fu Mai (Hidden)	Felt only on pressing hard to the bone		Syncope, severe pains, and retention of pathogenic factor in the interior of the body	
Lao Mai (Firm)	Felt firm, forceful, large, taut and long on pressing hard		Accumulation of Yin Cold and occurrence of masses	

The physiological deep pulse may be seen in people who are fat. The deep pulse may also be seen in winter because Yang Qi is deeply located.

C. Chi (slow), Huan (retarded)

- *Slow pulse (Chi Mai)*: This is slow in rate, with less than 4 beats per breath (less than 60 beats per minute). It indicates Cold syndromes. Because Cold makes Qi stagnated, Yang fails to do its transportation. A slow and forceful pulse means an Excess syndrome due to accumulation of Cold, while a slow and forceless ones means a Deficiency Cold syndrome.

- *Retarded pulse (Huan Mai)*: This is 4 beats per breath but has less strength in coming and going, which indicates Damp and deficiency of Spleen and Stomach. Because Damp is characterized by viscosity and stagnation, so Qi is disturbed in circulation. In cases where the Spleen and Stomach are deficient, Qi and Blood will be not sufficient to fill up the vessels, so the pulse is retarded.

Comparison

	Manifestations		Significance	
Chi Mai (Slow)	Less than 4 beats per breath (less than 60 beats per minute)	Slow and forceful	Cold syndromes	Excess Cold syndrome
		Slow and forceless		Deficiency Cold syndrome
	Slow and forceful pulse, tidal fever, abdominal fullness, constipation		Interior Excess Heat syndrome (Yangming Fu Excess syndrome)	
Huan Mai (Retarded)	4 beats per breath but less strong in coming and going	Retarded and forceless	Damp; deficiency of Spleen and Stomach	
		Even and forceful	A normal pulse with Wei (Stomach)	

The physiological slow pulse may be seen in athletes and people who are engaged long term in physical work.

D. Shu (rapid), Ji (swift)

- *Rapid pulse (Shu Mai)*: This is more than 5 beats per breath (more than 90 beats per minute) and indicates Heat syndromes. Because Heat makes Qi and Blood accelerate in circulation, it is a rapid and forceful pulse. In the case of prolonged disease, Yin deficiency gives rise to internal Heat, so it is rapid and forceless. If Yang is deficient, floating outside, the pulse will be rapid but forceless, feeling hollow on pressing.

- *Swift pulse (Ji Mai)*: This is swift, being 7–8 beats per breath, and indicates Yang hyperactivity and Yin exhaustion, and collapse of Yuan-primary Qi. Because the genuine Yin is exhausted in the inferior, the isolated Yang is hyperactive in the upper, and Qi is collapsed. When it is swift and hard this means a failure of exhausted Yin to control Yang, which is hyperactive. If it is swift and forceless this means primary Yang in collapse.

Comparison

	Manifestations		Significance	
Shu Mai (Rapid)	More than 5 beats per breath	Rapid and forceful	Heat syndromes	Excess Heat syndrome
		Rapid and forceless		Deficiency Heat syndrome
	Rapid but forceless, feeling hollow on pressing		Deficient Yang floating outside	
Ji Mai (Swift)	7–8 beats per breath	Swift and hard	Yang hyperactivity and Yin exhaustion, and collapse of Yuan-primary Qi	Failure of exhausted Yin to control Yang, which is hyperactive
		Swift and forceless		Primary Yang in collapse

The normal pulse of children is 5–6 beats per breath (about 100 beats per minute) and that of infants is 7–8 beats per breath (about 120 beats per minute). The pulse of healthy people can be quicker after physical exercises and in emotional excitation.

E. Xu (feeble), Shi (strong), Chang (long), Duan (short)

- *Feeble pulse (Xu Mai)*: This is weak and hollow at the Cun Guan Chi pulse points, and indicates deficiency of Qi and Blood and hypofunction of the Zang Fu organs. Because Qi is deficient in pushing Blood, so the pulse is weak; the Blood is deficient in filling the vessels, so the pulse is hollow.

- *Strong pulse (Shi Mai)*: This is forceful at Cun Guan Chi, and indicates Excess syndrome. Because pathogenic Qi is strong and antipathogenic Qi is not weak, the struggle between them is fierce, Qi and Blood are in excess and so the pulse is strong.

- *Long pulse (Chang Mai)*: This is straight and longer at Cun Guan Chi, and indicates Liver Yang excess and internal Heat due to excessive Yang. Because of excessive Liver Yang and internal Heat, the pulse is taut and extends longer.

- *Short pulse (Duan Mai)*: This is short in extent, and is distinct only at Guan, which indicates disorders of Qi. Short and forceful means Qi stagnation while short and forceless means Qi deficiency. Because deficiency of Qi is not able to push Blood, so the pulse is short and forceless; but stagnation of Qi with Blood stasis or retention of Phlegm Damp gives rise to obstruction of vessels, so the pulse is short and forceful.

Comparison

	Manifestations		Significance
Xu Mai (Feeble)	Weak and hollow at Cun Guan Chi		Deficiency – deficiency of Qi and Blood, hypofunction of Zang Fu organs
Shi Mai (Strong)	Forceful at Cun Guan Chi		Excess syndrome – pathogenic Qi strong and antipathogenic Qi not weak
Chang Mai (Long)	Straight and longer at Cun Guan Chi		Liver Yang excess, internal Heat due to excessive Yang
Duan Mai (Short)	Short in extent, distinct only at Guan	Short and forceful	Qi stagnation
		Short and forceless	Qi deficiency

Healthy people with sufficient Qi and Blood in circulation have the longer pulse, which is even and forceful.

F. Hong (surging), Da (large)

- *Surging pulse (Hong Mai)*: This is broad, large and forceful like roaring waves which come on powerfully and fade away, and indicates massive Heat in the Qi stage, because Heat makes vessels expand and Qi and Blood come powerfully. In the cases of prolonged disease, consumptive disease, strain, loss of Blood, and long-term diarrhoea, a surging pulse implies that the pathogen is strong and the antipathogenic Qi weak.

- *Large pulse (Da Mai)*: This is surging but without momentum of roaring waves. It indicates the progressive pathogens and antipathogenic Qi deficiency.

Comparison

	Manifestations		Significance	
Hong Mai (Surging)	Broad, large and forceful like roaring waves, which come on powerfully and fade away		Massive Heat in Qi level	
	Surging at superficial pressing, rootless at deep pressing		Prolonged disease with Qi deficiency, consumptive disease, strain, loss of Blood, long-term diarrhoea	
Da Mai (Large)	Surging but without momentum of roaring waves	Large rapid forceful	Pathogens progressing	Pathogenic Qi excess
		Large, forceless		Antipathogenic Qi deficiency

A physical surging pulse can be present in summer due to excessive Yang. A surging pulse but one that is even at all of Cun Guan Chi in a healthy person means strong antipathogenic Qi.

G. Xi (thready), Ru (thready soft superficial), Ruo (soft deep weak), Wei (thready soft feeble)

- *Thready pulse (Xi Mai)*: This is a fine thread but hits the finger distinctly and clearly, indicating deficiency of Qi and Blood, various other deficiencies, and diseases relating to Damp. Because Qi and Blood are deficient, the vessels are not filled up; because Qi is deficient in pushing Blood, the pulse is fine and weak as a soft thread; and the Damp blocks in the vessel.

- *Thready soft superficial pulse (Ru Mai)*: This feels superficial, fine and soft, hitting the finger without strength, indicating various deficiency and Damp disorders. Because the Essence and Blood are deficient, the vessels are not filled up, so the pulse is soft and weak. Because the Damp blocks in the vessels, so the pulse is without strength.

- *Soft deep weak pulse (Ruo Mai)*: This is very soft, deep and fine and indicates deficiency of Qi and Blood. The vessels are not filled up and hit the finger without strength.

- *Thready soft feeble pulse (Wei Mai)*: This is very fine and soft, and feels as though it has nearly vanished. It indicates deficiency of Yang, Qi, Yin and Blood. Owing to the deficiency of Yang Qi, the pulse has no power to hit the finger. It feels as if it has nearly vanished at gentle palpation because of the Yang Qi deficiency, while the feeling that it has nearly vanished at heavy palpation is because of Yin Qi exhaustion.

Comparison

	Manifestations	Significance
Xi Mai (Thready)	A fine thread hitting the finger distinctly and clearly	Deficiency of Qi and Blood, various other deficiencies, and diseases relating to Damp
Ru Mai (Thready soft superficial)	Superficial, fine and soft, hitting the finger without strength	Various deficiency and Damp disorders
Ruo Mai (Soft deep weak)	Very soft and deep and fine	Deficiency of Qi and Blood
Wei Mai (Thready soft feeble)	Very fine and soft, feeling like it is nearly vanished	Serious deficiency of Yang, Qi, Yin and Blood

In winter, when the weather is very Cold, the vessels are contracted, and the pulse feels deep and thready. A deep and thready pulse can also be present in fat people.

H. Hua (rolling), Dong (shaking), Se (hesitant)

- *Rolling pulse (Hua Mai)*: This feels smooth and flowing like pears rolling on a dish and indicates Phlegm and retained fluid, retention of food and excess Heat. Because the substantial pathogens cause excess of Qi and Blood, the pulse is rolling. It is usual in pregnant women and indicates the abundance and harmony of Qi and Blood.

- *Shaking pulse (Dong Mai)*: This feels like beans being shaken, beating rapidly and forcefully. It indicates pain and fright. Its presence is the result of Qi and Blood rushing due to Yin and Yang struggling, the vessels are shaking with Qi and Blood and the pulse is rapid and forceful. Pain comes from Qi stagnation and Blood stasis, fright causes disordered Qi and Blood and so the pulse shakes with discomfort.

- *Hesitant pulse (Se Mai)*: This feels rough, like a knife scraping on bamboo, and indicates damage of Essence, insufficiency of Blood, Qi stagnation and Blood stasis, retention of Phlegm and/or food. Because the insufficiency of Blood and Essence fails to nourish the vessels, Qi stagnation and Blood stasis give rise to a rough pulse. Qi stagnation causes Blood stasis in retention of Phlegm and/or food, and so the pulse is hesitant.

Comparison

	Manifestations		Significance
Hua Mai (Rolling)	Smooth and flowing like pears rolling on a dish		Phlegm fluid, retained fluid, retention of food, excess Heat
Dong Mai (Shaking)	Like beans being shaken, beating rapidly and forcefully, especially at Guan		Fear and fright, pain
Se Mai (Hesitant)	Rough like a knife scraping on bamboo	Forceful	Qi stagnation and Blood stasis, retention of Phlegm and/or food
		Forceless	Insufficiency of Essence and Blood

The presence of the rolling pulse in a pregnant woman means an abundance and harmony of Qi and Blood. A healthy person with a rolling pulse means his Ying-nutrient and Wei-defence are sufficient.

I. Xuan (string-taut), Jin (tense)

- *String-taut pulse (Xuan Mai)*: This feels taut, straight and long, shaped like a violin string, and indicates disorders of the Liver and Gallbladder, pain, Phlegm, and malaria. Because the stagnated pathogen in the Liver makes it disordered in keeping the free flow of Qi, the pulse is taut. Various pains and Phlegm retention make the vessels tense and the Qi in vessels blocked, so the pulse is taut.

- *Tense pulse (Jin Mai)*: This feels tight and forceful like a stretched rope, and indicates Cold, pain and retention of food. The pathogenic Cold struggling with Yang Qi causes spasm of vessels. If the pathogenic Cold is in the superficial part of the body, the pulse will be superficial and tight, while if the pathogenic Cold is deep in the body, the pulse will be deep and tight. The presence of a tense pulse in painful diseases and retention of food means that the pathogenic Cold is struggling with antipathogenic Qi.

Comparison

	Manifestations	Significance
Xuan Mai (String-taut)	Taut, straight and long, shaped like a violin string	Disorders of Liver and Gallbladder, pain, Phlegm, malaria
	String-taut and thready, like pressing on a knife edge	Disappearance of Stomach-Qi (critical sign of the pulse, symbolizing the decay of visceral energy)
Jin Mai (Tense)	Tight and forceful like a stretched rope	Excess Cold syndrome, pain, retention of food

A slight string-taut pulse can even be seen occasionally in spring in a healthy person, but the pulse of those in old age with hard vessels is always string-taut.

J. Cu (abrupt), Jie (knotted), Dai (intermittent)

- *Abrupt pulse (Cu Mai)*: This feels hurried, with irregular missed beats, and indicates excessive Yang Heat, stagnation of Qi and Blood, retention of Phlegm or food, and acute pyogenic infections. Because Yang excess with extreme Heat causes the failure of Yin to be harmonious with Yang, the pulse is hurried, with missed beats. A forceful abrupt pulse will be present in all excess Heat syndromes due to stagnation of Qi and Blood, retention of Phlegm and food, and acute pyogenic infections.

- *Knotted pulse (Jie Mai)*: This is slow with irregular missed beats, and indicates excessive Yin with Qi stagnation, Cold Phlegm with Blood stasis, and masses in the abdomen. Because Yin excess with Cold causes the failure of Yang to be harmonious with Yin, the pulse is slow with missed beats. A knotted pulse is present in the syndromes of Cold Phlegm with Blood stasis and Qi stagnation resulting in the obstruction of vessels.

- *Intermittent pulse (Dai Mai)*: This is slow with regular missed beats and indicates the decline of Zang Qi, Wind syndromes, painful syndromes, disorders due to emotional fear and fight, and traumatic injuries. Because of the decline in Zang Qi, insufficiency of Qi and Blood, and deficiency of Qi derived from the congenital Essence make the meridian Qi not continuous in circulation, the pulse has regular missed beats. In the Wind syndromes, painful syndromes, disorders due to emotional fear and fight, and traumatic injuries, the discontinuous circulation of meridian Qi is also the reason for the presence of intermittent pulse.

Comparison

	Manifestations		Significance
Cu Mai (Abrupt)	Hurried with irregular missed beats	Forceful	Excessive Yang Heat, stagnation of Qi and Blood, retention of Phlegm or food
		Fine, small, forceless	Exhaustion of Qi, Blood, and Yin
Jie Mai (Knotted)	Slow with irregular missed beats	Forceful	Excessive Yin with Qi stagnation, Cold Phlegm with Blood stasis, masses in abdomen
		Forceless	Exhaustion of Qi, Blood, and Yang
Dai Mai (Intermittent)	Slow with regular missed beats	Forceless	Exhaustion of Zang Qi
		Forceful	Bi syndromes, painful syndromes, disorders due to emotional factors, traumatic injuries

Comparison of 28 kinds of pulse

	Pulse	Manifestations	Significance
Superficial	Fu (Superficial pulse)	Easily felt with gentle touch, its strength slightly reduced but not hollow on a little heavy pressing	Exterior syndromes, Deficiency syndromes
	Hong (Surging pulse)	Broad, large and forceful like roaring waves that come on powerfully and fade away	Massive Heat
	Ru (Thready soft superficial pulse)	Thready, soft, superficial	Deficiency, Damp
	San (Scattered pulse)	Scattered, no roots, with fewer beats	Exhaustion of Yuan-primary Qi, failure of functions of Zang Fu organs
	Kou (Hollow pulse)	Floating, large, soft, hollow, like a scallion stalk	Severe loss of Blood, collapse of Yin
	Ge (Tympanic pulse)	Feels taut and hollow, as if touching the surface of a drum	Deficiency and Cold of Essence and Blood
Deep	Chen (Deep pulse)	Felt only on pressing hard	Interior syndromes
	Fu (Hidden pulse)	Felt only on pressing hard to the bone	Syncope, severe pains, retention of pathogenic factor in the interior of the body
	Lao (Firm pulse)	Firm, forceful, large, taut, long	Accumulation of Yin Cold, hernia, masses
	Ruo (Soft deep weak pulse)	Soft, deep, fine	Deficiency of Qi and Blood

	Pulse	Manifestations	Significance
Slow	Chi (Slow pulse)	Slow in rate with less than 4 beats per breath	Cold syndromes
	Huan (Retarded pulse)	4 beats per breath but less in strength	Damp syndromes, deficiency of Spleen
	Se (Hesitant pulse)	Rough like a knife scraping on bamboo	Damage of Essence, insufficiency of Blood, Qi stagnation and Blood stasis
	Jie (Knotted pulse)	Slow with irregular missed beats	Excessive Yin with Qi stagnation, Cold Phlegm with Blood stasis
Rapid	Shu (Rapid pulse)	More than 5 beats per breath	Heat syndromes, Deficiency syndromes
	Cu (Abrupt pulse)	Hurried with irregular missed beats	Excessive Yang Heat, stagnation of Qi and Blood
	Ji (Swift pulse)	Swift as 7–8 beats per breath	Yang hyperactivity and Yin exhaustion, collapse of Yuan-primary Qi
	Dong (Shaking pulse)	Like beans being shaken, rapid, forceful	Pain, fright
Feeble	Xu (Feeble pulse)	Weak and hollow	Qi and Blood deficiency
	Wei (Thready soft feeble pulse)	Very fine and soft, feeling as though it is nearly vanished	Deficiency of Yang, Qi, Yin and Blood, critical sign of Yang exhaustion
	Xi (Thready pulse)	As thin as a sewing thread, but hitting fingers clearly	Deficiency of Qi and Blood, Damp
	Dai (Intermittent pulse)	Slow with regular missed beat	Decline of Zang Qi, traumatic injury
	Duan (Short pulse)	Short in extent	Qi stagnation, Qi deficiency

Strong	Shi (Strong pulse)	Forceful at Cun Guan Chi	Excess syndrome
	Hua (Rolling pulse)	Smooth and flowing like pears rolling on a dish	Phlegm and retained fluid, retention of food, excess Heat
	Jin (Tense pulse)	Tight and forceful like a stretched rope	Cold, pain and retention of food
	Chang (Long pulse)	Straight and longer at Cun Guan Chi	Yang excess, internal Heat
	Xuan (String-taut pulse)	Straight, long, shaped like a violin string	Disorders of the Liver and Gallbladder, pain, Phlegm, malaria

K. Complicated pulse

The combination of two or more pulses present at the same time is known as a 'complicated pulse', and this indicates a combination of the indications of each single pulse.

Complicated pulse	Significance
Superficial tense (Fu Jin)	Exterior Cold syndrome, Bi syndrome
Superficial retarded (Fu Huan)	Exterior Deficiency syndrome (invasion of Wind to Taiyang)
Superficial rapid (Fu Shu)	Exterior Heat syndrome
Superficial rolling (Fu Hua)	Exterior syndrome combined with Phlegm – seen in those who with Phlegm generally are attacked by exogenous pathogenic factor
Deep slow (Chen Chi)	Interior Cold syndrome – Yang deficiency of Spleen and Stomach, stagnation of internal Cold
String-taut rapid (Xuan Shu)	Liver Heat syndrome – Liver-Qi stagnation transformed into Fire, Damp Heat of Liver and Gallbladder
Rolling rapid (Hua Shu)	Phlegm Heat, Phlegm Fire, internal Heat with retention of food
Surging rapid (Hong Shu)	Massive Heat in Qi stage – exogenous febrile disease
Deep string-taut (Chen Xuan)	Liver-Qi stagnation, retention of water fluid
Deep hesitant (Chen Se)	Blood stasis – Yang deficiency, Blood stasis due to Cold stagnation

Complicated pulse	Significance
String-taut thready (Xuan Xi)	Liver and Kidney Yin deficiency, Blood deficiency with Liver stagnation, Liver stagnation with Spleen deficiency
Deep retarded (Chen Huan)	Spleen deficiency, retention of water Damp
Deep thready (Chen Xi)	Yin deficiency, Blood deficiency
String-taut rolling (Xuan Hua)	Liver Fire combined with Phlegm, Wind Yang disturbing upward, accumulation of Phlegm and Fire

L. Female pulses

- *Menstruation pulse:*
  - The left Guan and Chi are suddenly big and stronger than those of the right, indicating that menstruation is coming.
  - Cun and Guan are normal, but Chi is weak thready hesitant, indicating unsmooth flow of menstruation.
  - Chi is weak thready hesitant, indicating amenorrhoea from a Deficiency syndrome.
  - Chi is wiry hesitant, indicating amenorrhoea from an Excess syndrome.

- *Pregnancy pulse:* Chi in particular is rolling rapid and smooth, accompanied by the cessation of menstruation together with preferences for a particular kind of food.

M. Infant pulse

- *Feeling method:* For a child less than 3 years old, the doctor holds the hand of the patient with his left hand, and puts his right thumb on the pulse of the child. For a child over 4 years old, the midpoint of the styloid process of the radius is taken as Guan. For a child more than 15 years old, the pulse is taken in the same way as for an adult.

- *Infant pulse:*
  - For children up to 3 years old, 7–8 beats within one breath is taken as the normal pulse.
  - 5–6 years old, 6 beats within one breath is the normal pulse, more than 7 beats is the rapid pulse and 4–5 beats is the slow pulse.

Only the superficial–deep, slow–rapid, and strong–weak of the infant pulse are observed, without consideration of other complicated conditions:

- Rapid indicates Heat while slow is Cold.

- Superficial and rapid are Yang while deep and slow are Yin.

- Strong–weak is to diagnose deficiency and excess.

- Deep and rolling mean the retention of food.

- Superficial and rolling show Wind Phlegm.

- Tense indicates Cold and retarded indicates Damp.

The favourable/deterioration case of a disease and diagnosis on the basis of symptoms or pulse condition

The favourable case of a disease refers to the compatibility of pulse and symptoms, while the deterioration case refers to the incompatibility of pulse and symptoms. However, a comprehensive analysis should be done using all of the four diagnostic methods, not simply following the pulse condition or symptoms.

2. PALPATION OF DIFFERENT PARTS OF THE BODY

The purpose of palpating the skin is to understand the cool–Heat and moist–Dry condition. Palpating the body and acupoints is done in order to understand the shape and size of masses. Palpating with pressure is to understand the tenderness, quality of a tumor, the severity of swelling and so on. The percussion method is used on the chest, abdomen and lumbus in order to understand the type of pain.

2.1 Palpating the skin

Signs			Significance	
Cool, prefer warmth			Cold syndrome	
Hot, prefer coolness			Heat syndrome	
Hot at the beginning but later not hot			Heat in the body surface	
Hot in long palpation, Heat from the inside to the body surface			Heat in the interior	
Burning hot of the body, cold limbs			True Heat with false Heat	
Oil-like sweating, warm limbs, rapid forceless pulse			Collapse of Yin	
Profuse Cold sweat, Cold skin, feeble pulse			Collapse of Yang	
Moist–dry	Moist		Sufficient Body Fluid, Qi and Blood	
	Dry, rough		Deficient Body Fluid, Qi and Blood	
	Scaly dry skin		Blood deficiency, Blood stasis	
Swelling	Depressed on pressure		Water swelling	
	Depressed on pressure but depression disappeared on removing pressure		Qi swelling	
Pain	Soft, prefer pressure		Deficiency syndrome	
	Hard, pain getting worse on pressure		Excess syndrome	
	Worse on pressure	Worse on mild pressure	Excess syndrome	Location of disease is shallow
		Worse on heavy pressure		Location of disease is deep

2.2 Palpating skin sores

	Signs	Significance
Sores	Local swelling, hardness, numbness, not hot	Cold syndrome
	Tenderness	Heat syndrome
	Flat root, diffuse swelling	Deficiency syndrome
	Higher than the skin	Excess syndrome
	Hard	No formation of pus
	Hard edges, soft top, feeling wave-like	Formation of pus

2.3 Palpating the hands and feet

	Signs	Significance
Cold and Heat	Cold hands and feet	Yang deficiency with Yin excess
	Hot hands and feet	Yang excess with Yin deficiency
	Hot dorsum of hands and feet	Fever in the exterior disease
	Hot palms and soles	Fever in the interior disease
Hot palms and forehead	Hot forehead	Exterior Heat
	Hot palms and soles	Interior Heat
Of an infant	Finger tips Cold	Convulsions
	Soles hot	Heat syndrome
	Legs Cold	Cold syndrome

2.4 Palpating the chest and abdomen

Xuli (the left costal region, between the fourth and fifth ribs) is palpated in order to understand the strength of Zong-pectoral Qi.

Xuli

Signs	Significance
The throbbing and rhythm of the heartbeat is not quick, nor slow, 4 to 5 beats one breath	Sufficiency of pectoral Qi
The slight throbbing does not hit the fingers clearly	Deficiency of pectoral Qi
The throbbing hits the patient's clothing	Outward going of pectoral Qi
Hitting the fingers strongly	Critical condition
Slow and weak throbbing, or rapid throbbing in the case of a weak constitution after a prolonged disease	Deficiency of Heart Yang
Feeble, without signs of death	Phlegm fluid
Strong throbbing without signs of dispersion	Excessive Heat

Chest and hypochondrium

Signs	Significance
Chest becoming higher, asthmatic breathing being induced on pressure	Lung distention
Distending pain in the chest and hypochondrium, solid sound on percussion	Pleural effusion
Hypochondriac pain getting better by pressure and becoming hollow on pressure	Liver deficiency
Mass in the hypochondrium, soft or hard	Qi stagnation of the Liver and Gallbladder with Blood stasis
Mass in the hypochondrium with an unsmooth surface	Liver cancer
Distending pain in the right hypochondrium, worse on pressure	Abscess of the Liver
Prolonged malaria with a mass in the hypochondrium	Malaria with splenomegaly

Abdomen

	Signs	Significance
Cold or Heat	Cold, prefer warmth and pressure	Deficiency Cold syndrome
	Hot, prefer Cold	Excess Heat syndrome
Pain	Pain, better on pressure	Deficiency syndrome
	Pain, worse on pressure	Excess syndrome
Burning pain, intolerable		Abscess of internal organs
Distention	Fullness and distention, feeling solid, with tenderness, heavy and turbid sound on percussion	Fullness of an excess
	Fullness, not solid when pressed, without tenderness, hollow sound on percussion	Fullness of a deficiency
Bulge of the whole abdomen	Extremely bulged as a drum, feeling like water in a bag when pressed, depression on the abdominal wall on pressure	Ascites
	As a drum on percussion, without the feeling of a water wave, no depression on the abdominal wall on pressure	Tympanites
Fullness in the epigastrium	Hard, tenderness, a resisting feeling on pressure	Excess syndrome
	Soft, no tenderness	Deficiency syndrome
	Distention, pain, with a watery sound on pushing	Fluid in epigastrium
Accumulation of Heat or Cold with stagnancy of fluid / Phlegm / Blood	Epigastric fullness, distention, and pain on pressure	Accumulation of Phlegm Heat in the chest
	Fullness and distending pain in chest, epigastrium and abdomen	Serious accumulation of Phlegm Heat in the chest

	Signs	**Significance**
Masses	Substantial mass with a fixed pain in abdomen	Accumulation in the Blood system
	Non-substantial mass with a moving pain in abdomen	Accumulation in the Qi system
	Hard nodules in the left lower abdomen	Faeces
	Nodules with pain on pressure in the right lower abdomen	Intestinal abscess
	Hard rope-like nodules like earthworms moving	Abdominal parasitosis

2.5 Palpating the acupoints

Palpating the acupoints to find nodules or rope-like objects, tenderness and other abnormal reactions can help diagnose the location of diseases.

- *Nodules at Feishu (BL13) or tenderness at Zhongfu (LU1)*: The disease is in the Lungs.

- *Tenderness at Ganshu (BL18) or Qimen (LV14)*: The disease is in the Liver.

- *Tenderness at Weishu (BL21) or Zusanli (ST36)*: The disease is in the Stomach.

- *Tenderness at Lanwei (EX-LE7)*: Intestinal abscess.

DIFFERENTIATION OF SYNDROMES

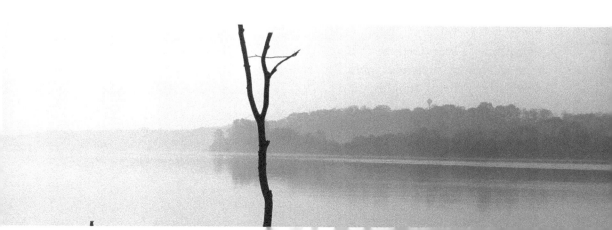

I. DIFFERENTIATION OF SYNDROMES ACCORDING TO THE THEORY OF THE EIGHT PRINCIPLES

CONCEPT OF DIFFERENTIATION OF SYNDROMES ACCORDING TO THE THEORY OF THE EIGHT PRINCIPLES

The Eight Principles are exterior and interior, Cold and Heat, deficiency and excess, Yin and Yang.

Differentiation of syndromes according to the Eight Principles is a method used to differentiate the location and nature of disease, and the relative strength of antipathogenic Qi and pathogenic factors on the basis of a comprehensive analysis of the data about the patient obtained using the four diagnostic methods.

In TCM, there are different methods for syndrome differentiation, and the differentiation of syndromes according to the Eight Principles is the most basic one. Any disease, in terms of its location, is exterior or interior; in terms of its nature, it is Cold or Hot, excess or deficiency, and in the category of Yin or Yang. Using differentiation in this way, the disease, no matter how complicated, can be recognized and diagnosed without difficulty.

1. EXTERIOR AND INTERIOR

Exterior and interior are the two principles that are used to determine the depth of the diseased area and to generalize the direction of the development of a disease.

Exterior syndrome: This refers to the pathological condition often seen in the early stage of exogenous diseases resulting from the invasion of the body surface by exogenous factors.

Interior syndrome: This refers to the pathological condition seen in the middle or late stage of a febrile disease or endogenous disease that has its diseased area in the interior (Zang Fu, Qi and Blood, bone marrow).

Exterior syndrome

Symptoms: Fever, aversion to Cold/Wind, headache, general aching, thin white tongue-coating, superficial pulse, accompanied with nasal obstruction, running nose, itching throat, cough.

Pathogenesis: Invasion of exogenous factors to the body surface blocks the Wei-defensive Qi, causing fever.

Analysis: Invasion of exogenous factors to the body surface blocks the Wei-defensive Qi, causing fever. The Wei-defensive Qi cannot warm the body surface, so there is an aversion to cold. Pathogenic factors stay in the meridians and collaterals, making Qi and Blood circulation obstructed, and thus causing a headache and general aching. Because the pathogenic factor is not yet transmitted to the inside, the tongue is not obviously changed. On invasion of the exogenous factor, the antipathogenic Qi comes to rest on the outside, so the pulse is superficial. The Lungs dominate the skin and skin hair, and the nose is the opening of the Lungs. The pathogenic factor enters from the skin, nose and mouth and into the Lungs, causing nasal obstruction, running nose, itching throat, and cough.

Characteristics: Sudden onset, short course, shallow location.

Key points: New disease, chills and fever, little change of tongue-coating, superficial pulse.

Interior syndrome

Symptoms: Complicated and varying with the different organs involved. High fever, irritability, coma, thirst, abdominal pain, constipation, diarrhoea, vomiting, scanty yellow urine, yellow or white thick sticky tongue-coating, deep pulse.

Pathogenesis: Inward transmitting of exogenous factors, direct invasion of exogenous factors to Zang Fu organs, emotional factors, improper diet, and overstrain and stress – dysfunction of the Zang Fu organs.

Analysis: Pathogenic Heat enters the interior, Cold is transformed into Heat and enters the interior, the internal Heat becomes strong leading to high fever. Heat consumes the Body Fluid, resulting in thirst, yellow scanty urine, and constipation. The pathogenic Heat disturbs the Mind stored in the Heart, leading to irritability and coma.

In the case of direct invasion of Cold to Zang Fu, or Cold Damp directly invading the Spleen and Stomach, because Cold is characterized by stagnation, then abdominal pain and diarrhoea are the result. The Stomach loses its normal descending function, leading to vomiting, yellow or white thick and sticky tongue-coating and deep pulse.

Characteristics: Slow onset, long course, deep location.

Key points: Fever with no chills, or chills with no fever, changes of tongue-coating, deep pulse, dysfunction of the Zang Fu organs.

Relationship between the exterior and interior syndromes

When exterior and interior are diseased simultaneously this is marked by exterior Cold with internal Heat, exterior Heat with interior Cold, exterior deficiency with interior excess, and exterior excess with interior deficiency.

As the pathogenic factor goes from the exterior to the interior, the disease is worse. For example, in the exterior syndrome, the patient has an aversion to cold and fever; if he then has an aversion to heat with thirst, he will have a preference for drinks, a red tongue with a yellow coating and yellow urine, indicating the inward movement of the pathogenic factor to the interior.

As the pathogenic factor goes from the interior to the exterior, the disease is relieved. For example, the patient has irritability, cough with a fullness in the chest, and then fever with sweating, or skin rashes, indicating the outward movement of the pathogenic factor to the exterior.

The intermediate syndrome, known as the half exterior and half interior syndrome, refers to the pathological condition in which the exogenous pathogenic factor fails to be transmitted completely to the interior, while the antipathogenic Qi is not strong enough to expel the pathogenic factor to the body surface. The pathogenic factor thus remains between the exterior and interior. The manifestations are alternating chills and fever, discomfort and fullness in the chest and hypochondrium, vomiting, anorexia, a bitter taste in the mouth, a dry throat, blurred vision and a wiry pulse.

2. COLD AND HEAT

Cold and Heat are the two principles that are used to differentiate the nature of the disease.

Cold syndrome: This refers to the pathological condition that results from exposure to exogenous pathogenic Cold or from deficiency of Yang in the interior of the body.

Heat syndrome: This refers to the pathological condition that is caused by invasion of exogenous pathogenic Heat or by deficiency of Yin in the interior of the body.

Cold syndrome

Symptoms: Aversion to Cold, preference for warmth, pale face, cold limbs, a lack of taste, absence of thirst, clear and thin Phlegm and nasal discharge, clear urine in increased volume, loose stools, pale tongue, with a white, moist coating, slow or tense pulse.

Pathogenesis: Invasion of pathogenic Cold, overeating of Cold and raw food, prolonged disease with Yang damaged, producing the internal Cold, Yang deficiency with excessive Yin.

Analysis: In Yang deficiency or invasion of Cold, Yang Qi is unable to warm the body, leading to cold limbs and pale face. Yin Cold is in the interior and Body Fluid is retained not consumed, leading to a lack of taste in the mouth and an absence of thirst. Water has failed to be transported and transformed when Yang is in deficiency, so there is clear and thin Phlegm and nasal discharge and clear urine in increased volume. The Spleen Yang is damaged by the Cold, with its normal function of transportation and transformation lost, leading to loose stools. The internal Cold Damp is produced by Yang deficiency, leading to pale tongue with a white, moist coating. Yang, if deficient, fails to promote the vessels for blood circulation, leading to a slow pulse. The pathogenic Cold is characterized by contraction, the vessels with Cold in them are contracted, and so there is a tense pulse.

Key points: Aversion to Cold, preference for warmth, pale face, absence of thirst, cold limbs, clear urine in increased volume, loose stools, pale tongue with a white, sticky coating, slow or tense pulse.

Heat syndrome

Symptoms: Aversion to Heat, preference for coolness, thirst with desire to have Cold drinks, red face and eyes, irritability, yellow and thick Phlegm and nasal discharge, haematemesis, epistaxis, yellow scanty urine, constipation, red tongue, with a yellow dry coating, rapid pulse.

Pathogenesis: Invasion of pathogenic Heat, Heat transformed from the Cold entering the interior, emotional stagnation transforming into Heat, retention of food accumulated into Heat, indulgence in sexual activities causing Yin Essence to be exhausted – Yang Heat excess, or Yin deficiency with internal Heat.

Analysis: Heat is preponderant, so there is an aversion to heat and a preference for coolness. The Body Fluid is consumed by the Heat, so there is yellow scanty urine and thirst, with a desire for Cold drinks. Fire is characterized by flaring up, so there is a red face and eyes. Heat disturbs the Mind stored in the Heart, leading to irritability. Heat consuming the Body Fluid causes yellow and thick Phlegm and nasal discharge. Fire burns the vessels, causing haematemesis and epistaxis. The Large Intestine is deprived of Body Fluid by Heat, leading to constipation. Red tongue and yellow dry coating indicate Heat syndrome. Heat accelerates the blood, leading to a rapid pulse.

Key points: Aversion to Heat, preference for coolness, thirst with desire to have Cold drinks, red face and eyes, hot limbs, constipation, yellow scanty urine, red tongue, yellow coating, rapid pulse.

Relationship between the Cold and Heat syndromes
A. Complicated syndromes of Cold and Heat

Heat above with Cold below: For example, the Heat above manifests as suffocation and Heat sensation in the chest with a desire to vomit; whilst the Cold below presents abdominal pain, which can be alleviated by warmth, and loose stools.

Cold above with Heat below: For example, the Cold above manifests as Cold pain in the epigastrium, with watery vomiting, and the Heat in the Bladder presents as frequent, painful urination with yellow scanty urine.

Exterior Cold with interior Heat: For example, aversion to cold, fever, no sweating, headache, general aching, asthmatic breathing, irritability, thirst, and superficial tense pulse.

Exterior Heat with interior Cold: For example, based on his constitutional weakness of Spleen and Stomach, the patient is attacked by pathogenic Wind Heat, thus suffers from fever, headache, cough, and sore throat, which are the manifestations of exterior Heat syndrome. At the same time, he has loose stools, clear urine in increased volume, and cold limbs, which are the symptoms of interior Cold syndrome.

B. Transformation of Cold and Heat syndromes

Cold syndrome transformed into Heat syndrome: In transformation of a Cold syndrome into Heat, the Cold syndrome occurs first and gradually changes into a Heat syndrome.

An example is exposure to exogenous pathogenic Cold, which may lead to an exterior Cold syndrome and produce aversion to cold, fever, white thin moist tongue-coating, and a superficial pulse. If this pathogenic Cold goes deep into the interior of the body and turns into Heat, the aversion to cold will subside, but there will be high fever, an aversion to heat, irritability, thirst, a red tongue with yellow coating and rapid pulse – that is, the symptoms of Heat syndrome will occur in succession.

Heat syndrome transformed into Cold syndrome: An example is that after profuse sweating or severe vomiting or diarrhoea, the body temperature of a high fever patient lowers abruptly, with the sudden appearance of cold limbs, pale complexion, and feeble pulse. This is the transformation of Heat syndrome into Cold.

C. True and false phenomena in Cold and Heat syndrome

True Cold with false Heat: For example, with the feverishness of the body, there is a flushed face, thirst, and a big pulse, looking like a Heat syndrome; however, the patient wants to cover up the body in spite of the feverishness, wants to have warm drinks to relieve the thirst, but does not drink much, and has a big pulse but forceless, cold limbs, watery diarrhoea, clear urine in increased volume, and a pale tongue with a white coating, which are the signs of Cold.

True Heat with false Cold: This is manifested as cold limbs and deep pulse, which are the signs of Cold syndrome, but the patient has no aversion to cold but has an aversion to heat, a deep rapid forceful pulse, accompanied with irritability, a thirst with preference for cold drinks, dry throat, foul breath, yellow scanty urine, constipation with dry stools, or dysentery of the Heat type, red tongue with a yellow dry coating – which reveal the true Heat of the disease.

Note: The false phenomena are usually seen on the limbs, skin and complexion. The truth should be taken from the interior, tongue and pulse for differentiation.

3. DEFICIENCY AND EXCESS

Deficiency and excess are the two principles that are used to generalize and distinguish the relative strength of the antipathogenic Qi and pathogenic factor.

Deficiency syndrome: This is pathological changes due to deficiency of antipathogenic Qi.

Excess syndrome: This is pathological changes due to invasion of pathogens, and caused by pathological products during the disease.

Deficiency syndrome

Symptoms: These include deficiency of Yin, Yang, Qi, Blood, Essence, and Body Fluid, and hypofunction of the Zang Fu organs.

These lead to: pallor, sallow complexion, listlessness, fatigue, palpitations, shortness of breath, cold limbs, spontaneous sweating, watery stools, incontinence of urine, a pale flabby tongue, a deep slow weak pulse, a hot sensation in palms and soles, emaciation, flushed cheeks, dry throat, tidal fever, night sweating, a red tongue with little coating, and a thready weak pulse.

Pathogenesis: Congenital deficiency, damage of acquired foundation (due to improper diet, emotional injuries, indulgence in sexual activities, or incorrect treatment damaging the antipathogenic Qi), including deficiency of antipathogenic Qi, malnutrition of Zang Fu organs, and a decline in physiological functions.

Analysis:

- *Damage of Yang*: Yang Qi is deficient, failing to warm and control, leading to pallor, cold limbs, listlessness, palpitation, shortness of breath, watery stools, incontinence of urine, a pale flabby tongue, and a deep slow weak pulse.

- *Damage of Yin*: Yin Blood is deficient, failing to control Yang, leading to a hot sensation in the palms and soles, irritability, palpitations, sallow complexion, flushed cheeks, tidal fever, and night sweating.

Excess syndrome

Symptoms: Fever, abdominal distention and pain, which are worse on pressure, coma, delirium, coarse breathing, Phlegm rattling in the throat, constipation, diarrhoea, tenesmus, scanty urine, painful urination, a tough tongue with a thick sticky coating, and an excessively forceful pulse.

Pathogenesis: Invasion of exogenous pathogenic factors, dysfunction of the Zang Fu organs resulting in Phlegm fluid, Water Damp, and Blood stasis. The pathogenic factors are strong, the antipathogenic Qi is not yet weak, as the struggle between the two is severe. There are the disorders of the functions of the Zang Fu organs.

Analysis: Hyperactivity of Yang Heat causes fever. Excess pathogen disturbs the Heart, causing irritability, coma and delirium. The dispersing function of the Lungs is injured, leading to fullness in the chest, coarse breathing, and Phlegm rattling in the throat. There is retention of the pathogen in the intestines, causing constipation and abdominal pain, which is worse on pressure. Downward affecting of Damp Heat leads to diarrhoea and tenesmus. There is retention of water Damp, disturbing the Qi activity of the Bladder leading to scanty urine. Damp Heat going to the Bladder produces painful urination. The struggle between the antipathogenic Qi and pathogenic factor in the vessels means that the pulse is forceful. Damp turbidity steams upward, so the tongue-coating is thick and sticky.

Differentiation

Deficiency syndrome

Qi:

- *Deficiency of Lung-Qi:* Asthmatic breathing, shortness of breath, spontaneous sweating, and low voice.

- *Deficiency of Qi of Middle Burner:* cold limbs, abdominal distention, abdominal pain, which is better on pressure, poor appetite, loose stools.

- *Deficiency of Yuan-primary Qi:* Flushing face, tinnitus, dizziness, palpitation, shortness of breath.

Blood:

- Pale lips and face, irritability, insomnia, listlessness, a deficiency of Body Fluid, night sweating, muscle spasm, and convulsions.

Zang:

- *Deficiency of Heart:* Sadness.

- *Deficiency of Liver:* Blurred vision, scrotum contraction, spasm of tendons, easily frightened.

- *Deficiency of Spleen:* Atrophy of limbs, indigestion, abdominal distention, worries.

- *Deficiency of Lungs:* Shortness of breath, skin without lustre.

- *Deficiency of Kidneys:* Dizziness, blurred vision, soreness and weakness in the lumbus and legs, constipation of a deficiency type, incontinence or retention of urine, seminal emission, diarrhoea at dawn.

Excess syndrome

Qi:

- *Excess of Lung-Qi:* Fullness in chest, dizziness and vertigo, profuse Phlegm with Qi retention in the chest causing a failure to lie down.

- *Excess of Stomach-Qi:* Fullness in the epigastrium, discomfort in the epigastric region, belching, acid regurgitation, vomiting, and hiccups.

- *Excess of Intestine Qi:* Abdominal distention, abdominal pain around the umbilicus, constipation, dysentery, tidal fever, and delirium.

- *Excess of Liver-Qi:* Headache, blurred vision.

Blood:

- *Blood stasis in skin and muscles*: Local blueness, swelling and pain.

- *Blood stasis in meridians and collaterals*: Aching of the body, spasm of tendons.

- *Blood stasis in Upper Burner*: Stabbing pain in chest, shoulder and arm.

- *Blood stasis in Middle Burner*: Epigastric and abdominal pain.

- *Blood stasis in Lower Burner*: Distention and stabbing pain in lower abdomen. Blood stasis causes a pain that is fixed or black stools.

Zang:

- *Excess of Heart*: Mental disorders, laughing all the time.

- *Excess of Liver*: Hypochondriac and abdominal pain, anger.

- *Excess of Spleen*: Abdominal distention, constipation, oedema.

- *Excess of Lungs*: Cough, abrupt breathing.

- *Excess of Kidneys*: Obstruction of Lower Burner, pain or distention.

A comprehensive analysis should be made for the diagnosis: Prolonged disease is mostly deficiency, while acute disease is usually excess. Attention should also be paid to the severity of the Cold and Heat and the changes in complexion, vitality, the nature of the pain, sweating, breathing, faeces and urine, tongue and pulse.

Relationship between the Deficiency and Excess syndromes
A. Complicated deficiency with excess

Excess with deficiency

Symptoms	Pathogenesis	Characteristics
In the case of invasion of exogenous Cold, the Phlegm Damp in the Stomach causes the Stomach-Qi to be damaged after the treatment of sweating, emetic, and purgation, with the symptoms of fullness in epigastrium and belching	In the process of Excess syndrome, the antipathogenic Qi is damaged; or people with a weak constitution are attacked by a pathogen	Excess pathogen is the primary, and the deficiency of antipathogenic Qi is the secondary characteristic

Deficiency with excess

Symptoms	Pathogenesis	Characteristics
In the case of Kidney Yin deficiency in a spring febrile disease, the pathogenic Heat damages the Liver and Kidney Yin, the pathogen in the late stage decreases and the antipathogenic Qi is seriously weakened. The symptoms are low fever, dry mouth, and dry dark red tongue	The antipathogenic Qi is seriously damaged in a prolonged Excess syndrome and the pathogenic factor has not yet been dispelled completely. Or people with constitutional deficiency get the invasion of pathogenic Qi	The deficiency of antipathogenic Qi is the primary, and excess pathogen is the secondary characteristic

Deficiency and excess

Symptoms	Pathogenesis	Characteristics
Retention of food in an infant damages the Spleen and Stomach with symptoms such as diarrhoea with undigested food in the stools, abdominal bulging, emaciation, irritability in the afternoon, a thick tongue-coating, and a thready and a bit of a wiry pulse	Antipathogenic Qi is seriously damaged in a prolonged serious Excess syndrome, but the pathogenic factor has not yet been reduced. Or people with weak antipathogenic Qi are attacked by a serious pathogenic factor	Both the deficiency of antipathogenic Qi and excess pathogen are serious, and therefore the pathological condition is serious

B. Transformation of excess and deficiency

In the process of a disease, the Excess syndrome can be transformed into a Deficiency syndrome when the antipathogenic Qi is damaged. Or, when pathological products are formed due to a dysfunction of the Zang Fu organs, the Deficiency syndrome will change into an Excess syndrome.

For example, an Excess Heat syndrome with high fever, thirst, sweating and surging pulse which is not properly treated will change into a Deficiency syndrome, with the manifestations of emaciation, a withered face, shortness of breath, a coatingless tongue, and a thready forceless pulse due to exhaustion of the Body Fluid.

C. True and false phenomena in deficiency and excess

True deficiency with a false excess refers to a syndrome of the deficiency type which is accompanied by symptoms and signs similar to a syndrome of excess type, and is known as 'extreme deficiency shows excess-like symptoms'.

True excess with false deficiency refers to a syndrome of excess type which is accompanied by symptoms and signs similar to a syndrome of deficiency type, and is known as 'big excess shows deficiency-like symptoms'.

Differentiation

Points that need to be established in order to make differentiation clear are as follows:

- whether the pulse is forceful or not, with or without Shen-vitality, superficial or deep
- whether the tongue is tender or tough
- whether the voice is low or loud
- whether the constitution is weak or strong
- what the pathogenic factors are
- the course of the disease
- the earlier treatment.

These should be all taken into consideration for diagnosis.

True deficiency with false excess

Pathogenesis	Symptoms	
Hypofunction of Zang Fu organs, deficiency of Qi and Blood, obstruction of Qi activity	False	Abdominal distention and pain, abrupt breathing, difficulty in discharging stools
	True	Abdominal distention becoming better on pressure, and without mass being felt, shortness of breath, stools not dry
	Accompanying symptom	Prolonged disease, listlessness, pale tongue, weak pulse

True excess with false deficiency

Pathogenesis	Symptoms	
Retention of pathogenic excess, Qi and Blood obstruction, deprived of nourishment and moisture	False	Depressed without talking, diarrhoea, tiredness, slim figure, deep thready pulse
	True	Loud voice, coarse breathing, getting relieved after discharging of stools, tired but feeling better with movement, epigastric and abdominal pain that is better on pressure, thready but forceful pulse
	Accompanying symptom	Dark tongue with Blood spots on it

4. YIN AND YANG

Yin and Yang form a pair of principles used to generalize categories of syndromes.

Plain Questions states: 'An experienced doctor differentiates Yin and Yang first when he observes and palpates the patient.'

Yin syndrome: Interior, Cold, Deficiency syndromes.

Yang syndrome: Exterior, Heat, Excess syndromes.

Yin syndrome

Symptoms: Dark complexion, listlessness, curved lying, cold limbs, no thirst, stools with a fishy smell, clear and increased volume of urine, a pale flabby tender tongue, and a deep slow weak thready hesitant pulse.

Pathogenesis:

- *Deficiency syndrome*: Pale dark complexion, listlessness, tiredness, low voice.

- *Interior Cold syndrome*: Cold limbs, no thirst, loose stools with bad smell, clear and increased volume of urine.

- *Deficiency Cold syndrome*: Pale flabby tender tongue, deep slow or thready hesitant pulse.

Analysis: Listlessness, tiredness and low voice indicate a Deficiency syndrome. cold limbs, no thirst, loose fish-smelling stools, clear and increased volume of urine indicate an interior Cold syndrome. A pale flabby tender tongue, a deep slow weak thready hesitant pulse are the signs of a deficiency Cold.

Yang syndrome

Symptoms: Red face, fever, hot skin, restlessness, loud voice, coarse breathing, abrupt breathing with Phlegm gurgling in the throat, thirst, stinking stools, yellow scanty urine, dark red tongue, burnt black thorny coating, superficial rapid surging rolling forceful pulse.

Pathogenesis:

- *Heat syndrome*: Red face, fever, hot skin, restlessness, thirst.

- *Excess syndrome*: Loud voice, coarse breathing, abrupt breathing with Phlegm gurgling in the throat, constipation with stinking stools, scanty yellow urine.

- *Excess Heat syndrome*: Dark red tongue, burnt black thorny coating, superficial rapid surging rolling forceful pulse.

Analysis: Red face, restlessness, hot skin and thirst indicate Heat syndrome. Loud voice, abrupt breathing, Phlegm gurgling in the throat, and constipation indicate Excess syndrome. Dark red tongue, burnt black thorny coating, and surging rolling forceful pulse indicate Excess Heat syndrome.

Differentiation

	Yin syndrome	Yang syndrome
Inspection	Pale dark complexion, lying in a curved position, tiredness, listlessness, pale flabby tender tongue, moistened slippery coating	Red face, hot skin, restlessness, dry mouth, dark red or black thorny tongue, dry yellow coating
Auscultation and olfaction	Low voice, inactive in talking, weak respiration, shortness of breath	Loud voice, talkative, coarse breathing, abrupt breathing with Phlegm rattling in throat, mania
Inquiring	Fishy stools, tastelessness, poor appetite, no thirst or preferring hot drinks, increased or scanty urine	Constipation with dry and stinking stools, anorexia, dry mouth, thirst, scanty yellow urine
Palpation	Abdominal pain that is better on pressure, Cold skin, deep weak thready hesitant slow pulse	Abdominal pain that is worse on pressure, hot skin, superficial surging rapid big rolling forceful slow pulse

A. Real Yin deficiency, Real Yang deficiency

Real Yin deficiency: Kidney Yin deficiency.

Real Yang deficiency: Kidney Yang deficiency.

	Real Yin deficiency	Real Yang deficiency
Symptoms	Emaciation, hot sensation in palms and soles, steaming Heat in bones, tidal fever, flushed cheeks, night sweating, irritability, insomnia, dizziness, tinnitus, yellow scanty urine, constipation, red tongue, little coating, thready rapid pulse	cold limbs, lying in a curved position, sleepiness, listlessness, shortness of breath, dislike of talking, pale complexion, spontaneous sweating, no thirst or preferring hot drinks, clear and increased volume of urine, loose stools, or with undigested food in the stools, pale flabby tongue, white slippery coating, deep slow weak pulse
Pathogenesis	With Yin deficiency, the internal Heat is produced, depriving Zang Fu of nourishment	With Yang deficiency, the internal Cold is produced, causing the failure of Yang to warm, transport and transform, and control

B. Collapse of Yin, Collapse of Yang

Collapse of Yin: Pathological conditions resulting from massive consumption of Yin fluid.

Collapse of Yang: Pathological conditions caused by extreme exhaustion of Yang Qi in the body.

Collapse of Yin	Collapse of Yang
Hot salty sweat, red face, warm limbs, red dry tongue, surging forceful rapid pulse which is forceless when pressed, restlessness, delirium, hot skin, coarse breathing, thirst with preference for Cold drinks	Cold sweat, pale face, cold limbs, white moistened tongue, superficial rapid hollow or feeble pulse, dull expression or coma, Cold skin, feeble breathing, no thirst, preference for hot drinks
Prolonged disease with an extreme Yin deficiency, high fever, serious sweating, vomiting, diarrhoea, big loss of Blood – exhaustion of Yin fluid, deficiency Fire in the inside, malnutrition of the Zang Fu organs	Prolonged disease with an extreme Yang deficiency, serious damage of Yang Qi by excessive Yin Cold, serious sweating, big loss of Blood. Yang is vanished in the exhaustion of Yin – collapse of Yang, accumulation of Yin Cold in the inside, hypofunction of the Zang Fu organs

Relations between the syndromes

A. Relationship between Cold-Heat and exterior-interior

Symptoms

Exterior Cold syndrome	Exterior Heat syndrome	Interior Cold syndrome	Interior Heat syndrome
Severe chills, mild fever, headache, general aching, no sweating, white moist tongue-coating, superficial tense pulse	Fever, slight aversion to Wind and Cold, headache, dry mouth, slight thirst, or sweating, red tongue tip and borders, superficial rapid pulse	cold limbs, pale complexion, no thirst, or preference for hot drinks, inactive in talking, clear and increased volume of urine, loose stools, pale tongue, white moist tongue-coating, deep slow pulse	Red face, hot skin, thirst, irritability, preference for Cold drinks, restlessness, talkative, yellow urine, constipation, red tongue with yellow coating, rapid pulse

Pathogenesis

Exterior Cold syndrome	Exterior Heat syndrome	Interior Cold syndrome	Interior Heat syndrome
Invasion of Cold damaging Wei-defence Yang, dysfunction of the Lungs in dispersing and descending	Invasion of Heat, Wei-defence Qi being obstructed	Direct invasion of Cold to Zang Fu, or deficiency of Yang Qi	Internal Heat consuming the Body Fluid

Analysis

Exterior Cold syndrome	Exterior Heat syndrome	Interior Cold syndrome	Interior Heat syndrome
Pathogenic Cold damages Wei-defence Yang, which fails to warm the body surface, leading to chills. In the struggle between the antipathogenic Qi and pathogenic factor, Yang Qi is obstructed, leading to fever. Cold stagnated in the vessels, causing headache and general aching. Cold is characterized by contraction, the skin pores are closed, leading to superficial tense pulse	Invasion of pathogenic Heat causes the Wei-defence Qi to be blocked, leading to fever and chills. Heat is a Yang pathogenic factor, so there is severe fever and mild chills, dry mouth and slight thirst. Heat is characterized by upward and outward movement, the skin pores opening, leading to sweating. Heat affects upward, leading to headache. Heat stays in the exterior, leading to red tongue tip and borders, and superficial rapid pulse	The direct invasion of Cold damages Yang Qi, which fails to warm the body, leading to cold limbs and pale complexion. Yin Cold is in the inside without damaging Body Fluid, so there is no thirst, or thirst with a preference for hot drinks. Yin Cold creates hypofunction, resulting in little talking. Clear urine and loose stools, pale tongue with white moist coating, and deep slow pulse are the signs of interior Cold	The interior Heat steams the skin, leading to red face and hot skin. Body Fluid is damaged, leading to thirst with a preference for Cold drinks. Yang Heat creates hyperfunction, causing restlessness with active talking. Body Fluid is damaged by Heat, leading to scanty yellow urine. The Body Fluid of the intestines is damaged, leading to dry stools. Red tongue with yellow coating and rapid pulse are the signs of interior Heat

B. Relationship between Deficiency-Excess, exterior-interior and Cold-Heat syndromes

Exterior Deficiency syndrome

	Symptoms	Pathogenesis	Analysis
Exogenous exterior Deficiency syndrome	Headache, stiff neck, fever, sweating, aversion to Wind, superficial pulse that is a bit slow	Invasion of Wind, disharmony between Ying-nutrient and Wei-defence	Wind obstructs the Taiyang Meridian, leading to a headache and stiff neck. Yang Qi goes outward and upward, leading to fever. Body surface is loose, with the skin pores opened by the Wind, leading to sweating and aversion to Wind. Wind stays on the body surface, so the pulse is a bit slow
Endogenous exterior Deficiency syndrome	Spontaneous sweating, and frequent catching Cold, accompanied by pale complexion, shortness of breath which is worse on exertion, tiredness, poor appetite, loose stools, pale tongue, white coating, thready weak pulse	Qi deficiency of the Lungs and Spleen, Wei-defence weakness	The Lungs dominate the skin and hair and the Spleen dominates the muscles. When Qi is deficient, the body surface becomes weak with unconsolidation of Wei-defence, leading to spontaneous sweating. Wei-defence is weak in protection, leading to frequent catching of Cold. Pale complexion, shortness of breath which is worse on exertion, tiredness, poor appetite, loose stools, pale tongue, white coating, thready weak pulse are due to Qi deficiency of the Lungs and Spleen

Exterior Excess syndrome

Symptoms	Pathogenesis and analysis
Symptoms of exterior syndrome and no sweating, general aching, superficial tense pulse	In invasion of Cold, Yang Qi comes to the body surface, struggling with the pathogenic Qi, the body surface is strong and pores are closed. Seen in the exterior Cold syndrome

Interior Deficiency syndrome

Symptoms	Pathogenesis	Analysis
Interior Deficiency Cold syndrome is of Yang Deficiency syndrome, manifested as cold limbs, lying in a curved position, sleepiness, listlessness, tiredness, shortness of breath, being inactive in talking, pale complexion, spontaneous sweating, no thirst, preference for hot drinks, clear and increased volume of urine, loose stools, with undigested food in the stools, pale flabby tongue, white slippery coating, deep slow forceless pulse	With Yang Qi deficiency, internal Cold is produced, causing the failure of warming, Qi activities and controlling. Same as that in the deficiency Cold syndrome	Same as that in the Deficiency Cold syndrome

Interior Excess syndrome

	Symptoms	Pathogenesis	Analysis
Interior Excess Cold syndrome	Cold pain that is alleviated by warmth, pale complexion, cold limbs, abdominal pain that is made worse by pressure, cough with Phlegm rattling in the throat, salivation, clear and increased volume of urine, white moist tongue-coating, slow or tense pulse	Preponderance of internal Cold results in obstruction of Yang Qi	Pathogenic Cold blocks Yang Qi, producing Cold pain that is better on warmth, and cold limbs. Stagnation of Cold blocks the meridians and collaterals, causing abdominal pain that is worse on pressure. Yang Qi in deficiency is unable to nourish the face, so there is a pale complexion. Cold makes the Spleen low in transportation and transformation owing to the disturbance of Spleen Yang, leading to borborygmus and diarrhoea. Cold attacks the Lungs, producing cough and Phlegm, salivation, clear and increased volume of urine, and white moist tongue-coating. Cold makes the Blood circulation slow, so slow pulse
Interior Excess Heat syndrome	High fever, thirst, preference for Cold drinks, red face and eyes, restlessness, coma, delirium, abdominal distention and pain that is worse on pressure, constipation, yellow scanty urine, red tongue, yellow dry coating, surging rolling rapid forceful pulse	Internal Heat consumes the Body Fluid	The internal Heat is strong, leading to high fever. Fire flares, leading to red face and eyes. Heat disturbs the Mind stored in the Heart, leading to restlessness, coma and delirium. Heat stagnates in the intestines, leading to abdominal distention and pain that is worse on pressure, and constipation. Yin fluid is consumes by Heat, causing yellow scanty urine, thirst, and preference for Cold drinks. Red tongue and yellow coating indicates Heat inside. Heat is likely to disturb the Blood and vessels, leading to a surging rolling rapid forceful pulse

Deficiency Cold syndrome

Symptoms	Pathogenesis	Analysis
Listlessness, pale complexion, cold limbs, abdominal pain which is better on pressure, loose stools, clear and increased volume of urine, tiredness, pale tender tongue, weak deep slow pulse	With Yang Qi deficiency, internal Cold is produced, causing the failure of warming, Qi activities and controlling. Same as that in the interior deficiency Cold syndrome	With Yang Qi deficiency, the function of Qi is weak, leading to listlessness, a pale complexion, tiredness, pale tender tongue, and weak deep slow pulse. Without the warmth of Yang Qi, the manifestations will be cold limbs, abdominal pain that is better on pressure, loose stools, and clear and increased volume of urine

Deficiency Heat syndrome

Symptoms	Pathogenesis	Analysis
Flushed cheeks, emaciation, tidal fever, night sweating, hot sensation in palms and soles, dry throat, red tongue, little coating, thready rapid pulse	Deficiency of Yin fluid, production of deficiency Heat, malnutrition of Zang Fu	Exhaustion of Yin fluid produces emaciation, tidal fever and night sweating. Deficiency Fire flares up, causing flushed cheeks, dry throat, red tongue and little coating. Yin Blood is deficient, leading to a thready pulse. Deficiency Heat inside leads to thready rapid pulse

II. DIFFERENTIATION OF SYNDROMES ACCORDING TO THE THEORY OF AETIOLOGY

The purpose of the differentiation of syndromes according to the Theory of Aaetiology is to identify the causative factors of diseases by analysing the clinical manifestations, which is known as 'seeking the causative factors by differentiating symptoms and signs'.

1. DIFFERENTIATION OF SYNDROMES ACCORDING TO THE THEORY OF THE SIX EXOGENOUS FACTORS AND PESTILENTIAL EPIDEMIC FACTORS

1.1 Differentiation of syndromes according to the Theory of the Six Exogenous Factors

Wind

Symptoms: Fever, aversion to Wind, headache, sweating, cough, obstruction of nose, running nose, thin white tongue-coating, superficial retarded pulse, or numbness of limbs, spasm of tendons, convulsions, opisthotonus, itching.

Pathogenesis: Wind is the leading causative factor of many diseases. It is characterized by upward and outward dispersion. The disorders caused by Wind are marked by migratory symptoms, rapid changes and abrupt onset of diseases.

Analysis: The invasion of Wind damages the defensive Qi and makes the body surface weak, leading to fever, an aversion to Wind, headache, and sweating. Wind damages the Lungs in dispersing, leading to a cough, obstruction of the nose, and a running nose. A thin white tongue-coating and superficial retarded pulse indicate the invasion of Wei-defence by Wind. The body surface is attacked by Wind, leading to numbness. Wind attacks the meridians and collaterals, causing spasm in tendons, convulsions, and opisthotonus. Itching is the symptom of Wind affecting the skin.

Key points: Aversion to Wind, sweating, itching throat, superficial pulse, itching, urticaria, abnormal movement of limbs and rapid changes of symptoms.

Cold

Symptoms: Aversion to Cold, fever, no sweating, headache, aching of the body, cough, thin white tongue-coating, spasm of limbs, cold limbs, feeble pulse, abdominal pain, borborygmus, diarrhoea, vomiting.

Pathogenesis: Cold is a Yin pathogenic factor, characterized by contraction and stagnation, damaging Yang Qi and obstructing Qi and Blood.

Analysis: Invasion of Cold obstructs Wei-defence Qi, which is not able to disperse, leading to an aversion to cold, fever, and no sweating. Cold stagnates in the meridians, leading to headache and aching of the body. The skin is attacked, involving the Lungs which then fail in dispersing, leading to cough and obstruction of the nose. There is an invasion of Cold to the body surface, leading to a superficial tense pulse and a thin white tongue-coating. Yang Qi is damaged by the Cold stagnated in the meridians, thus causing spasm of the limbs. With the Cold, Yang Qi cannot move into the limbs, leading to cold limbs; without the warmth of Yang Qi, there is also a feeble pulse. Cold invades the interior, damaging the Spleen and Stomach, producing disorders in transportation and transformation, leading to abdominal pain, borborygmus, diarrhoea, and vomiting.

Key points: Aversion to Cold, cold limbs, Cold pain, preference for warmth, pale tongue, white slippery coating.

Summer Heat

Symptoms: When one is attacked by Summer Heat, there is an aversion to heat, sweating, thirst, tiredness, yellow urine, red tongue, with a yellow or white coating, and a weak rapid pulse.

In the case of sunstroke, there is fever, falling down in a fit with a loss of consciousness, sweating, thirst, abrupt breathing, convulsions, a dark red dry tongue, and a soft thready rapid pulse.

Pathogenesis: Pathogenic Summer Heat is characterized by upward movement, dispersion and consumption of Body Fluid. It is frequently combined with pathogenic Damp.

Analysis: If attacked by Summer Heat, Qi and Body Fluid are consumed, leading to an aversion to heat, sweating, thirst and yellow urine. Because of sweating, Qi is exhausted, resulting in tiredness and a weak rapid pulse. An invasion of Summer Heat combined with Damp attacking the Upper Burner, leads to a yellow or white coating of the tongue. In sunstroke, the Summer Heat disturbs the Mind stored in the Heart, leading to a falling down in a fit with a loss of consciousness. Summer Heat consumes Qi and Body Fluid, leading to fever, sweating, thirst, and abrupt breathing. The Pericardium is disturbed by Summer Heat and Damp, leading to a loss of consciousness. Exhaustion of Qi and Body Fluid stirs up the Liver Wind, leading to convulsions. Summer Heat damages Ying Yin, leading to a dark red dry tongue and a soft thready rapid pulse.

Key points: Seen in summer. The weather is hot, and so Qi and Body Fluid are consumed by Heat.

Damp

Symptoms: Distending pain in the head, fullness in chest, lack of thirst, heaviness and pain of the body, fever, tiredness, clear and increased volume of urine, a white slippery tongue-coating, and a soft thready retarded pulse. Headache with a sensation as if the head is wrapped in bandages, tiredness of limbs, a soft thready weak pulse, and painful heavy joints with motor impairment.

Pathogenesis: Pathogenic Damp is characterized by heaviness and viscosity. Damp diseases are long in duration.

Analysis: Damp is likely to damage the skin, muscles, and tendons. The pathogenic condition with heavy and painful joints and motor impairment caused by pathogenic Damp is known as 'fixed Bi'.

Key points: Heaviness of the body, fullness in the epigastrium, turbid and large amount of excretion, thick sticky tongue-coating, prolonged course of disease, relating to humid environment and rainy weather.

Dryness

Symptoms: Cool dryness: slight headache, aversion to cold, no sweating, cough with itching in the throat, obstruction of the nose, a dry tongue, and a superficial pulse.

Warm dryness: Feverish sensation in the body, sweating, thirst, dry throat, cough, chest pain, Blood-tinged sputum, dry nose, dry tongue, yellow coating, superficial rapid pulse.

Pathogenesis: Pathogenic dryness, including warm dryness and cool dryness, consumes the Body Fluid.

Analysis:

- *Cool dryness*: In the late stages of autumn, the weather is Cold and dry. If the Lung is attacked by cool dryness, the symptoms will be a slight headache, aversion to cold, no sweating, cough, nasal obstruction, itching throat, dry tongue, and superficial pulse.

- *Warm dryness*: In the early stage of autumn, it is still quite hot. If the Lungs are attacked by warm dryness, there will be a feverish sensation in the body, sweating, thirst, a dry throat, cough, dry nose, and Blood-tinged sputum.

Key points: Seen in autumn with the symptoms of dry nose, mouth, throat and skin, unproductive cough or a little sticky sputum that is difficult to spit out. The manifestations of exterior syndrome are present at the same time.

Fire

Symptoms: High fever, thirst, red face and eyes, restlessness, delirium, spitting Blood, epistaxis, skin rashes, mania, pus formation, dark red tongue, surging rapid or thready rapid pulse.

Pathogenesis: Fire is burning in nature and consuming the Body Fluid. It causes stirring of Wind due to tendons and muscles being deprived of moisture. Pathogenic Fire disturbs Blood by accelerating its circulation.

Analysis: Pathogenic Fire burns the Qi system, resulting in high fever, thirst, red face and eyes, and surging pulse. Heat enters the Blood, accelerating its circulation and causing extravasation, leading to spitting of Blood, epistaxis, and skin rashes. Fire burns the Heart and Liver, leading to mania. Fire damages muscles, leading to pus formation. Dark red tongue and thready rapid pulse indicate that Fire goes deep into the Blood.

Key points: Fever, aversion to heat, red face, irritability, thirst with desire for drinks, mania, bleeding, local redness, swollen, hotness and pain with pus formation, dark red tongue, yellow and dry coating.

1.2 Differentiation of syndromes according to the Theory of the Pestilential Epidemic Factors

Pestilential epidemic factors cause severe infectious diseases characterized by sudden onset and rapid transmission.

Epidemic febrile disease

Symptoms: At the beginning, the patient has an aversion to cold and later fever, and then a fever without aversion to cold. In the first 2–3 days, he has rapid pulse, headache, general aching, afternoon fever, and a thick white tongue-coating.

Pathogenesis: An infectious epidemic disease is caused by a pestilential factor and characterized by sudden onset with a critical condition.

Analysis: The pathogenic factor in the pleuro-diaphragmatic interspace affects the Wei system, producing chills and fever and aching of the body. An accumulation of pathogens causes a thick white powder-like tongue-coating. The head is the convergence of all Yang meridians. When Fire flares up and burns the Body Fluid, Heat steams to the head, leading to sweating of the head.

Epidemic eruption

Symptoms: Fever, headache as if the head is splitting, red or purple or black eruptions, rapid pulse.

Pathogenesis: An eruptive disease caused by a pestilential factor.

Analysis: The pestilential factor invades via the skin, mouth and nose to the Lungs and Stomach, then to all 12 meridians, causing fever, headache, and eruptions. Rapid pulse indicates the pestilential Heat steaming.

Fulminant jaudice

Symptoms: At the beginning, there is fever and aversion to cold, then quickly the whole body, including the teeth and eyes, become dark yellow in colour. In severe cases, there are Cold extremities, unconsciousness, delirium, staring eyes, enuresis, shrinking of the tongue, and an involuntary movement of fumbling and picking at the bed or clothes.

Pathogenesis: Fulminant jaundice is a pathological condition caused by a pestilential factor in combination with Damp Heat.

Analysis: A pestilential factor in combination with Damp Heat affects the skin and muscles, leading to an aversion to cold, a fever and a sudden change of the whole skin of the body to dark yellow. A pestilential factor enters the Zang Fu organs, and so Yin and Yang are not connected with each other, causing cold limbs. When pestilence disturbs the Mind stored in the Heart, coma and delirium occur. The upward movement of the pathogen disturbs the brain, causing staring eyes. The downward movement of the pathogenic factor causes the disorder of the Lower Burner, leading to enuresis and scrotum contraction. The pestilential factor invades the interior of the Zang organs, exhausting the Essence and Qi, leading to shrinking of the tongue and involuntary movements of fumbling and picking at the bed or clothes.

Developing direction of disease

To the outside: Being agitated, sweating after shivering, spontaneous sweating.

To the inside: Fullness in chest and epigastirum, distending pain in abdomen, constipation, accumulation of dry faeces in the Large Intestine with discharge of foul water, vomiting, coma, delirium, yellow tongue, black thorny coating.

2. DIFFERENTIATION OF SYNDROMES ACCORDING TO THE THEORY OF THE SEVEN EMOTIONAL FACTORS

The seven emotional factors are: joy, anger, melancholy, worry, grief, fear and fright. Severe, continuous or abruptly occurring emotional stimuli that surpass the regulative adaptability of the organism will affect the physiological functions of the human body, especially when there is a pre-existing oversensitivity to them. The Qi and Blood of the Zang Fu organs will be disturbed, leading to disease.

	Symptoms	Pathogenesis
Joy	Irritability, incoherent speech, abnormal behaviours	The Heart-Qi is slack, leading to incoherent speech
Anger	The Liver-Qi is perverted and the Blood is abnormally rising, leading to sudden syncope	Anger damages the Liver. The disordered Liver-Qi leads to the Blood going up abnormally
Melancholy	Mental depression, listlessness, poor appetite	Melancholy and worry damage the Lungs, and Qi is obstructed, leading to mental depression. When the Spleen is involved in a prolonged case, there will be poor appetite
Worry	Forgetfulness, palpitations, poor sleep, emaciation	Over-thinking damages the Spleen; with the Heart involved, the symptoms will be palpitations, forgetfulness, insomnia, and emaciation
Grief	Pale complexion, listlessness	Grief damages the Qi of the Lungs, which dominates the Qi of the whole body. When the Lungs are damaged, Qi vanishes, leading to a pale complexion
Fear	Frightened and restless	Fear damages the Kidneys, causing Kidney-Qi deficiency
Fright	Restlessness, mental disorders, abnormal speaking and behaviours	Fright makes Qi disordered, disturbing the Mind stored in the Heart, leading to restlessness and mental disorders

Key point for differentiation

The Heart, Liver and Spleen are mainly involved. People experiencing many emotional stimuli or who have uncommunicative dispositions or psychological defects are easily affected. Disease symptoms can get better or become worse as a result of the emotional changes.

3. IMPROPER DIET, OVERSTRAIN, STRESS

Improper diet

Symptoms: If the Stomach is damaged there will be epigastric pain, poor appetite, fullness in the epigastrium, acid regurgitation, a thick, sticky tongue-coating, and a rolling forceful pulse.

If the intestines are damaged, there will be abdominal pain and diarrhoea.

Retention of food produces a rolling rapid or deep forceful pulse and a yellow, thick, sticky tongue-coating.

Pathogenesis: Improper diet damages the Stomach, the Qi of which is disordered and therefore does not descend, so there is poor appetite, epigastric pain, and fullness in the epigastrium. The functions of the intestines are disturbed by the retention of food, and there will be abdominal pain and diarrhoea. When the food retention is in the Middle Burner, the Qi of which is obstructed, there will be a rolling rapid or deep forceful pulse. The retained food and the Stomach Turbid Qi mix with each other and steam upward, leading to a thick sticky tongue-coating and foul breath.

Overstrain, stress and lack of physical exercise

Symptoms: Overstrain and stress result in tiredness, sleepiness, inactivity in talking, poor appetite, and a retarded big or superficial or thready pulse.

A lack of physical exercise causes obesity, asthmatic breathing that is worse on exertion, palpitations, shortness of breath, and weakness of limbs.

Pathogenesis: Overstrain and stress damage Yuan-primary Qi, leading to tiredness and sleepiness.

A lack of physical exercise causes obstruction of Qi circulation, following which there will be unsmooth Blood circulation, leading to palpitations and shortness of breath.

Sexual indulgence

Symptoms: Yin deficiency produces cough with bloody sputum, steaming Heat in bones, afternoon fever, palpitations, and night sweating.

Yang deficiency produces impotence, prospermia, cold limbs, soreness and weakness in palms and soles, nocturnal emissions and spermatorrhoea.

Pathogenesis: Yin deficiency with Yang hyperactivity means Fire flares and Phlegm is formed, resulting in steaming Heat in bones and afternoon fever.

Yang deficiency causes the lack of consolidation of sperm, leading to nocturnal emissions and spermatorrhoea. Tendons and muscles lack nourishment leading to impotence, soreness and weakness in palms and soles, and cold limbs.

4. TRAUMATIC INJURY

Traumatic injury includes gunshot wounds, incisions, contusions, scalds, burns, sudden contracture or sprains due to carrying heavy loads, and insect or animal bites. Muscular swelling and pain, Blood stasis, bleeding, damage of tendons, fracture of bones, dislocation of joints, toxicosis, etc., which are due to traumatic injury can, in severe cases, result in damage to internal organs, causing loss of consciousness or even death.

	Symptoms	Pathogenesis
Soft tissues	Local pain, swelling, blue skin	Injury of tendons and muscles – Qi stagnation and Blood stasis
Body surface	Skin wounds, bleeding, pain	Injury of collaterals
Fracture, joint dislocation	Local swelling and pain, motor impairment	Joints and bones damaged by violent force
Injury of Zang Fu and vessels	Local pain, bleeding, dysfunction of Zang Fu, or even dyspnoea, loss of consciousness, and death	Injury of Zang Fu organs and vessels – broken Zang Fu with dysfunctions, Qi collapsed with bleeding

Key points for differentiation

History of trauma, local pain with motor impairment, image examination if necessary.

III. DIFFERENTIATION OF SYNDROMES ACCORDING TO THE THEORY OF QI, BLOOD AND BODY FLUID

1. SYNDROMES OF QI

Deficiency of Qi: Pathological changes resulting from hypofunction of Zang Fu organs.

Sinking of Qi: Pathological changes that develop from a deficiency of Qi.

Stagnation of Qi: Pathological changes when Qi in a certain part of the body or a specific Zang Fu organ is retarded and obstructed.

Perversion of Qi: Pathological changes occurring with dysfunction of the Qi in ascending and descending.

Deficiency of Qi

Symptoms: Shortness of breath, dislike of speaking, lassitude, dizziness, blurred vision, spontaneous sweating, which is worse on exertion, pale tongue with a white coating, weak pulse.

Pathogenesis: Prolonged diseases, overwork, weak constitution in old age.

Analysis: Deficiency of Yuan-primary Qi causes hypofunction of the Zang Fu organs, leading to shortness of breath, a dislike of speaking, and lassitude. Clean Yang fails to ascend due to Qi deficiency, leading to dizziness and blurred vision. The body surface is weak and pores open, leading to spontaneous sweating, which is worse on exertion. Blood does not go up to nourish the tongue in the case of Qi deficiency, leading to a pale tongue with a white coating. The Blood circulation is weak, resulting in a weak pulse.

Key points: Hypofunction of the Zang Fu organs.

Sinking of Qi

Symptoms: Shortness of breath, dizziness, blurred vision, prolonged diarrhoea, bearing-down sensation and distention in abdomen, and prolapse of rectum or uterus.

Pathogenesis: This develops from Qi deficiency or damage of the Qi in a certain Zang Fu organ due to overwork; Qi is too weak to go up, and so sinks.

Analysis: Qi is deficient, leading to dizziness, blurred vision, shortness of breath, a pale tongue with a white coating, and a weak pulse. Qi of the Middle Burner is deficient, sinking down, leading to prolonged diarrhoea and gastroptosis with a bearing-down sensation and distention in the abdomen. Ptosis of the Liver and Kidneys causes a bearing-down sensation in the hypochondrium and lower abdomen. Prolapse of uterus occurs in the female with the sinking of Qi.

Key points: Bearing-down sensation in abdomen, prolonged diarrhoea, ptosis and symptoms of Qi deficiency.

Stagnation of Qi

Symptoms: Fullness and distention, pain.

Pathogenesis: Caused by retention of pathogenic factors, emotional stagnation, and Yang deficiency with which the Zang Fu organs are lacking warmth and Qi circulation is obstructed.

Analysis: Distention, pain, onset or made worse by emotional factors.

Key points: Fullness and distention plus pain.

Perversion of Qi

Symptoms: Cough, asthma, hiccup, belching, nausea, vomiting, dizziness, headache, syncope, haematemesis.

Analysis:

- *Perversion of Lung-Qi*: Cough, asthma.
- *Perversion of Stomach-Qi*: Hiccup, belching, nausea, vomiting.
- *Perversion of Liver-Qi*: Dizziness, headache, syncope, vomiting.

Key points: Perversion of Qi of Lungs and Stomach, or over-dispersing of Qi of Liver.

2. SYNDROMES OF BLOOD

Deficiency of Blood: Zang Fu organs lacking nourishment, leads to hypofunction of the whole body.

Stagnation of Blood: Extravasated Blood forms Blood stasis, and is obstructed in vessels and Zang Fu organs.

Heat in the Blood: Fire accelerating Blood.

Cold in the Blood: Cold stagnating Blood.

Deficiency of Blood

Symptoms	Pathogenesis	Analysis	Key points
Pale or sallow complexion, pale lips and nails, insomnia, palpitations, numbness of limbs, scanty menstrual flow which is light in colour, amenorrhoea, pale tongue with white coating, thready weak pulse	Congenital deficiency, weakness of Spleen and Stomach in producing Qi and Blood, bleeding, prolonged disease, and overthinking can cause exhaustion of Blood; or Blood stasis in the body inhibits the production of new Blood	There is a lack of nourishment causing a pale or sallow complexion, pale lips and nails. Brain and eyes have a poor Blood supply leading to dizziness and blurred vision. The Heart is deprived of Blood for carrying out its normal function, leading to insomnia and palpitations. Meridians and collaterals are short of nourishment from Blood deficiency, leading to numbness of limbs. Menstrual flow, lacking Blood because of Blood deficiency, is scanty or ceases	Pale skin all over the body plus weakness of the whole body

Stagnation of Blood

Symptoms	Pathogenesis and Analysis	Key points
Stabbing fixed pain, worse at night and on pressure	The pathogenic factor obstructs the Blood circulation, causing pain. The Blood stagnation gets worse at night, leading to pain getting worse. Mostly seen in cases with perversion of Lung and Stomach-Qi or over-dispersing of Liver-Qi	Stabbing pain fixed in the local area, worse at night and on pressure plus masses, purple lips and nails and thready hesitant pulse
Masses: On skin, the skin is blue. In abdomen, the mass is hard and fixed	Blood stasis forms the mass	
Repeated bleeding, dark in colour, blood clots, black stools	Blood stasis obstructs blood circulation, making the blood vessels break and causing bleeding. The extravasated blood flowing out causes bleeding, and staying within the body becomes the causative factor of subsequent bleeding	
Dark face, rough skin, purple lips and nails, subcutaneous bleeding, blue veins on the surface of the abdomen seen clearly, distending pain in lower limbs on which the blue veins are seen clearly	Retention of Blood stasis obstructs the blood circulation, depriving the skin and nails of nourishment	
Purple dark tongue, blue skin, thready hesitant pulse	Signs of Blood stasis	
Amenorrhoea, dysmenorrhoea	Retention of Blood stasis, no production of new blood	

Heat in the Blood

Symptoms	Pathogenesis	Analysis	Key points
Haemoptysis, haematemesis, bloody urine, epistaxis, dark red tongue, wiry rapid pulse	Overwork, over-drinking of alcohol, anger damaging the Liver, accumulation of Heat due to sexual indulgence. Heat entering Blood	Fire of Zang Fu forces blood to be extravasated, causing bleeding. Blood Heat produces a wiry forceful pulse	Bleeding plus signs of Heat

Cold in the Blood

Symptoms	Pathogenesis	Analysis	Key points
Pain of hands and feet, dark Cold hands and feet which are better with warmth, Cold pain in lower abdomen, cold limbs, late menstruation, menstrual Blood dark in colour and with clots. Dark tongue with white coating, deep slow hesitant pulse	Invasion of Cold	Cold in Blood causes pain of hands and feet, dark Cold hands and feet which are better in warmth. Cold in uterus causes a Cold pain in lower abdomen, and cold limbs. The menstrual flow is disturbed by Cold, which causes Blood stasis, leading to its dark colour and presence of clots. Qi and Blood are not circulated to the upper part due to Cold stagnation, causing a dark tongue with a white coating. Deep pulse indicates interior syndrome; slow pulse indicates Cold syndrome, and hesitant pulse indicates Blood stasis	Cold pain in a local area, which is better on warmth, dark tongue, white coating, deep slow hesitant pulse

3. SYNDROMES OF QI AND BLOOD

Qi stagnation and Blood stasis: The syndrome of Blood stasis caused by an obstruction of Qi circulation.

Qi deficiency and Blood stasis: The syndrome of Blood stasis caused by a deficiency of Qi.

Deficiency of both Qi and Blood: The syndrome developed from deficiency of both Qi and Blood.

Failure of Qi in controlling Blood: The bleeding due to Qi deficiency.

Collapse of Qi in bleeding: The bleeding that produces the collapse of Qi.

Qi stagnation and Blood stasis

Symptoms	Pathogenesis	Analysis	Key points
Distending pain in hypochondrium, hot temper, hypochondriac masses with a stabbing pain that is worse on pressure, amenorrhoea, dark menstrual flow with clots, dark purple tongue, hesitant pulse	Mental depression and Liver-Qi stagnation are the causative factors	Liver-Qi stagnation causes distending pain in the hypochondrium. The Liver loses its normal function in keeping Qi free-flowing, causing hot temper. The Blood stasis due to prolonged Qi stagnation causes hypochondriac masses. Obstruction of Qi circulation produces a stabbing pain that is worse on pressure. The Qi stagnation makes the menstrual flow irregular, causing amenorrhoea or dysmenorrhoea. Dark purple tongue and hesitant pulse are the signs of Blood stasis	Prolonged course, pain in the distributing areas of the Liver Meridian, masses, symptoms of Qi stagnation and symptoms of Blood stasis

Qi deficiency and Blood stasis

Symptoms	Pathogenesis and analysis	Key points
	Qi becomes deficient in a prolonged disease, producing Blood stasis	Symptoms of Qi deficiency plus symptoms of Blood stasis
Pale or dark complexion, lassitude, shortness of breath, inactive in talking	Qi deficiency makes blood circulation slow, causing a pale or dark complexion	
Stabbing pain fixed in hypochondrium and worse on pressure, dark tongue with Blood spots, deep hesitant pulse	Obstruction of Blood causes a stabbing pain that is worse on pressure. Seen mostly in Heart and Liver diseases, so the pain is in the chest and hypochondrium. Deep pulse indicates the interior syndrome and hesitant pulse indicates Blood stasis	

Deficiency of both Qi and Blood

Symptoms	Pathogenesis and analysis	Key points
	Qi becomes deficient, unable to produce new Blood	Symptoms of Qi deficiency plus symptoms of Blood deficiency
Shortness of breath, inactive in talking, tiredness, spontaneous bleeding	Qi deficiency of the Lungs and Spleen is the cause	
Dizziness, blurred vision, pale or dark complexion, palpitation, insomnia, pale tender tongue, thready weak pulse	The Heart is lacking in Blood, causing palpitations and insomnia. Blood deficiency causes the vessels to empty, causing a pale or dark complexion, pale tender tongue, and thready weak pulse	

Failure of Qi in controlling Blood

Symptoms	Pathogenesis and analysis	Key points
	Prolonged disease causes Qi deficiency, and Qi is exhausted with chronic bleeding. In turn, the deficiency of Qi causes bleeding	Bleeding plus symptoms of Qi deficiency
Haematemesis, haematochezia, subcutaneous bleeding, functional uterine bleeding	Qi is deficient, unable to control Blood	
Pale complexion, pale tongue, thready weak pulse	Blood deficiency is the cause	

Collapse of Qi in bleeding

Symptoms	Pathogenesis and analysis	Key points
	Trauma, damage of internal organs, delivery, functional uterine bleeding	In a major loss of Blood, the occurrence of Qi collapse is seen
With serious loss of Blood, there is a sudden onset of pale face, cold limbs, profuse sweating, or even syncope, pale tongue, feeble pulse, or floating big and slack pulse	Yang Qi collapses when it loses its ability to hold Blood in place during major bleeding, causing a pale face, cold limbs, profuse sweating, or even syncope. The tongue loses its Blood supply and the vessels have no Blood to fill them, causing a pale tongue and feeble pulse. Yang Qi floats outward and vanishes, causing a floating big and slack pulse	

4. SYNDROMES OF BODY FLUID

4.1 Deficiency of Body Fluid

The whole body or a certain Zang Fu organ loses moisture.

Symptoms	Pathogenesis	Analysis	Key points
Dry mouth, lips, nose, tongue, throat, and skin, scanty urine, dry stools, red dry tongue, thready rapid pulse	Insufficient production – weakness of Spleen and Stomach. Severe loss – Heat consuming Body Fluid, sweating, vomiting, diarrhoea	In exhaustion of Body Fluid, the Zang Fu and skin lose moisture, causing scanty urine and dry stools. In a deficiency of Body Fluid, Blood formation is decreased, causing a red dry tongue and a thready, rapid pulse	Dry mouth, lips, nose, tongue, throat, and skin, scanty urine, dry stools

4.2 Retention of Water

A. Oedema

Retention of Water causing oedema of face, limbs, chest and abdomen or even the whole body.

Yang oedema: Oedema of an excess type.

Yin oedema: Oedema of a deficiency type.

Yang oedema

Symptoms	Pathogenesis	Analysis
Oedema starting from the head and eyelids and then moving to the whole body, the skin looking thinner and bright, scanty urine, accompanied with aversion to Wind, fever, thin white tongue-coating, superficial tense pulse, or sore throat, red tongue, superficial rapid pulse	Invasion of pathogenic Wind	The Lungs lose their function in dispersing, descending and regulating the Water passage. The Water fluid is disordered in distribution, flowing to the skin. The Wind and Water combines to form the oedema, known as the 'syndrome of Wind and Water in combination'

Key points: Sudden onset, starting from eyelids and face, oedema of the upper part of body more serious than that of the lower part, fever, aversion to Wind, aching of the body, sore throat, superficial pulse

Yin oedema

	Symptoms	Pathogenesis and analysis
		Prolonged disease causing the deficiency of antipathogenic Qi, overwork, overindulgence in sexual activities
Oedema with a depression of skin on pressure, pale complexion, scanty urine	Oedema especially below the lumbus, accompanied with fullness in chest, abdominal distention, poor appetite, loose stools, listlessness, heaviness of the body, pale tongue, white slippery coating, deep pulse	Water is not well transported and transformed by the Spleen, going downward, so oedema starts from the feet and is especially severe in lower part of the body. The Middle Burner is out of its normal function in transportation and transformation, causing fullness in chest, abdominal distention. Retention of water causes a pale face, listlessness, heaviness of the body, and a white slippery tongue-coating. A deep pulse indicates the interior syndrome
	Oedema gets worse day by day, accompanied with soreness and weakness in lumbus and knees, scanty urine, cold limbs, pale flabby tongue, with a white slippery coating and a deep slow weak pulse	Kidney Yang is damaged by the Spleen deficiency, so the oedema gets worse day by day. The Qi activity of the Bladder is not normal, causing scanty urine. In Kidney Yang deficiency, the body is not warmed, leading to soreness and weakness in the lumbus and knees, and cold limbs. Water is flourishing when Kidney Yang is deficient, causing a pale flabby tongue with a white slippery coating, and a deep slow weak pulse

Key points: Repeated attacks and a long course of oedema, starting from the feet; oedema of the lower part of the body is more serious than that of the upper part

B. Phlegm fluid

Phlegm syndrome: The pathological condition in which the thick part of Water, Tan-Phlegm, stays in the Zang Fu organs, meridians and collaterals, and between tissues.

Fluid syndrome: The pathological condition in which the thinner part of Water, Yin-fluid, stays in the Zang Fu organs and between tissues.

Phlegm syndrome

Symptoms	Pathogenesis
Phlegm	Dysfunctions of Zang Fu caused by invasion of the six exogenous factors, and emotional factors
Cough with Phlegm, asthma, fullness in chest	Retention of Phlegm in the Lungs, Qi of the Lungs rising
Fullness in epigastric region, poor appetite, nausea, watery vomiting, dizziness, blurred vision	Phlegm staying in the Stomach, Qi of the Stomach rising
Loss of consciousness, mania, Phlegm rattling in throat	Phlegm misting the Heart produces mental disorders
Numbness of limbs, hemiplegia, scrofula, foreign body sensation in the throat, nodules in breast	Phlegm staying in meridians and collaterals or subcutaneous region, and muscles causing irregular Blood circulation, producing the MeiheQi in the throat
White sticky or yellow sticky tongue-coating, rolling pulse	Sticky tongue-coating and rolling pulse indicate the retention of Phlegm turbidity

Fluid syndrome

Symptoms	Pathogenesis
Yin	Dysfunctions of Zang Fu is the cause
Cough, asthma, fullness in chest, thin and profuse amount of Phlegm, Phlegm rattling in throat, unable to lie flat (excessive fluid in the hypochondrium and epigastrium)	Fluid staying in the Lung, Qi of the Lungs rising
Fullness and distention in epigastrium and abdomen, watery sound in intestines, watery vomiting, poor appetite (Phlegm retention)	Fluid staying in the Stomach and Intestines, Qi of the Stomach rising
Fullness and distending pain in chest and hypochondrium, cough bringing on the pain (pleural effusion)	Fluid staying in chest and hypochondrium, Qi circulation getting blocked
Palpitations, dizziness, cold limbs, oedema of the lower extremities	Fluid affecting the Heart, Yang of the Heart is obstructed
White slippery tongue-coating, wiry pulse	Fluid, being a Yin pathogenic factor, is manifested in a wiry pulse

IV. DIFFERENTIATION OF SYNDROMES ACCORDING TO THE THEORY OF THE ZANG FU ORGANS

The differentiation of syndromes of the Zang Fu organs is a method used to analyze the location and nature of disease and the relative strength of antipathogenic Qi, and pathogenic Qi according to the physiological functions and pathological changes of the Zang Fu organs.

1. SYNDROMES OF THE HEART AND SMALL INTESTINE

Diseases of the Heart

Pathological changes:

1. The Heart's control of the Blood and blood vessels fails, and so disturbance of Blood circulation is present.

2. The Heart's housing of the Mind becomes disordered and so abnormal mental activities appear.

Symptoms: Palpitations, irritability, cardiac pain, insomnia, dream-disturbed sleep, forgetfulness, delirium.

Deficiency syndromes: Deficiency of Heart-Qi, deficiency of Heart Yang, sudden collapse of Heart Yang, deficiency of Heart Blood, deficiency of Heart Yin.

Excess syndromes: Hyperactivity of Heart Fire, Phlegm misting the Heart, Phlegm Fire disturbing the Heart.

Ben-deficiency Biao-excess syndromes: Obstruction of the Heart vessels.

Diseases of the Small Intestine

Pathological changes: The Small Intestine's separation of the clear from the turbid becomes abnormal.

Symptoms: Painful urination, bloody urine.

Excess syndromes: Excess Heat of the Small Intestine.

1.1 Deficiency of Heart-Qi, deficiency of Heart Yang, sudden collapse of Heart Yang

Deficiency of Heart-Qi: Weakness of the Heart-Qi in circulating the Blood is indicated by a group of Qi deficiency symptoms, with palpitations as the main one.

Deficiency of Heart Yang: Insufficiency of Heart Yang in warming the interior is symptomized by a group of symptoms of Deficiency Cold syndrome.

Sudden collapse of Heart Yang: Extreme deficiency of Heart Yang develops into sudden collapse of Yang.

The three conditions have the following symptoms in common: palpitations, fullness in the chest, shortness of breath, spontaneous sweating.

Deficiency of Heart-Qi

Symptoms: Listlessness and lassitude that become worse on exertion, pale complexion, pale tongue with white coating, weak pulse.

Pathogenesis: Deficiency of Heart-Qi.

Analysis: Deficiency of Heart-Qi causes lassitude, pale complexion, pale tongue, and weak pulse.

Deficiency of Heart Yang

Symptoms: Cardiac pain, aversion to cold, cold limbs, pale swollen tongue with white watery coating, thready feeble pulse.

Pathogenesis: Heart-Qi deficiency develops into Heart Yang deficiency, which fails to warm the interior and thus produces the deficiency Cold there.

Analysis: Heart-Qi deficiency plus symptoms of deficiency Cold.
   Obstruction of Heart vessels causes cardiac pain. Yang deficiency fails to warm and circulate Blood, producing thready forceless pulse.

Sudden collapse of Heart Yang

Symptoms: Sudden onset of cardiac pain, profuse Cold sweat, cold limbs, feeble breathing, pale complexion, cyanosis of lips, coma (purplish tongue, feeble fading pulse).

Pathogenesis: Heart Yang deficiency develops into sudden collapse of Heart Yang.

Analysis: Heart Yang deficiency plus symptoms of collapse of Yang.

Heart Yang deficiency causes cold limbs and profuse Cold sweating. The weak pectoral Qi fails to help the Lungs in respiration, leading to feeble breathing. The collapsed Yang causes the Blood to stagnate in the vessels, presenting as pale complexion and cyanosis of lips. The Mind stored in the Heart is deprived of nourishment, leading to coma.

1.2 Deficiency of Heart Blood, deficiency of Heart Yin, hyperactivity of Heart Fire

Deficiency of Heart Blood: Symptoms of Blood deficiency due to poor nourishment of the Heart.

Deficiency of Heart Yin: Symptoms of restlessness of the Mind stored in the Heart due to deficiency Heat.

These two conditions have the following symptoms in common: palpitations, insomnia, dream-disturbed sleep. The Heart is lacking nourishment, leading to palpitations. The Mind stored in the Heart is deprived of nourishment, causing insomnia and dream-disturbed sleep.

Hyperactivity of Heart Fire: Symptoms of excess Heat disturbing the Mind due to the Heart Fire.

Deficiency of Heart Blood

Symptoms: Dizziness, forgetfulness, pale complexion, pale lips, pale tongue, thready and weak pulse.

Pathogenesis: Palpitations, insomnia, forgetfulness plus symptoms of Blood deficiency.

Analysis: The brain marrow is poorly nourished, causing dizziness and forgetfulness. The Blood deficiency causes pale complexion, pale lips, and pale tongue. The vessels are not filled up, resulting in a thready and weak pulse.

Deficiency of Heart Yin

Symptoms: Hot sensation in the Five Centres, afternoon fever, flushed cheeks, red tongue with little coating, thready rapid pulse.

Pathogenesis: Palpitation, irritability, insomnia, dream-disturbed sleep, forgetfulness plus symptoms of Yin deficiency.

Analysis: Yin deficiency gives rise to Yang hyperactivity. The internal Heat causes hot sensation in the Five Centres and afternoon fever. The deficiency Fire flares up, causing flushed cheeks and a red tongue with little coating. A thready pulse is caused by Yin defiency and a rapid pulse by Heat.

Hyperactivity of Heart Fire

Symptoms: Irritability, insomnia, delirium, redness of face, thirst, yellow urine, dry stools, dark red tongue tip, ulcers of tongue, rapid forceful pulse, or spitting Blood, epistaxis, redness, hotness and painful skin with sores.

Pathogenesis: The emotional stagnation is transformed into Fire, or an invasion of Heat or prolonged over-intake of rich food, indulgence in drinking alcohol or smoking results in transformation of Fire.

Analysis: Irritability, insomnia, delirium, ulcers of the tongue, dark red tongue tip plus symptoms of interior excess Heat
   The Mind stored in the Heart is disturbed by Heat, leading to irritability, insomnia, and delirium. The internal Heat causes redness of the face, thirst, yellow urine, dry stools, and a rapid forceful pulse. The Heart Fire flares up, causing a dark-red tongue tip and ulcers of the tongue. The hyperactive Heart Fire forces the Blood to accelerate, causing spitting of Blood and epistaxis.

1.3 Obstruction of the Heart vessels

This refers to those syndromes with the manifestations of obstruction of Heart vessels caused by Blood stasis, Phlegm, Yin Cold, Qi stagnation, etc.

Symptoms: Palpitations, cardiac pain which is often referred to the shoulder and arm.

Pathogenesis and analysis: The Heart Yang is not active, the Heart lacks warmth and nourishment, leading to palpitations. The Heart Blood is not circulated well because of the Yang deficiency, causing cardiac pain. The Heart Meridian runs upward to the Lungs and comes out from the axillary fossa and goes along the medial side of the arm, and so the pain is felt in the shoulder and arm.

	Symptoms	Pathogenesis and analysis
Blood stasis in Heart vessels	Stabbing pain in precordial region, dark tongue with Blood spots on it, thready hesitant pulse or intermitant pulse	Stabbing pain in precordial region plus symptoms of Blood stasis
Phlegm in Heart vessels	Fullness and pain in precordial region, profuse Phlegm, heaviness and tiredness of the body, white and sticky tongue-coating, deep rolling or hesitant pulse	Fullness and pain in precordial region plus symptoms of Phlegm
Cold in Heart vessels	The precordial pain becomes worse with Cold while it is relieved by warmth. cold limbs, pale tongue with white coating, deep slow or tight pulse	Cold pain in the precordial region plus symptoms of interior Cold
Qi stagnation in Heart vessels	Distending pain in precordial region, hypochondriac distention, sighing, light red tongue, string-taut pulse	Distending pain in the precordial region plus symptoms of Qi stagnation

1.4 Phlegm misting the Heart, Phlegm Fire disturbing the Heart

Phlegm misting the Heart: This is manifested as disorder of mental activities since the Mind is disturbed by Phlegm.

Phlegm Fire disturbing the Heart: This is manifested as disorder of mental activities since the Mind is disturbed by Fire and Phlegm.

These two syndromes have the following symptoms in common: mental disorders, fullness in the epigastric region, profuse Phlegm, sticky tongue-coating, rolling pulse.

Phlegm misting the Heart

Pathogenesis and analysis: Mental disorders plus symptoms of Phlegm turbidity.
Invasion of Damp blocks the Qi circulation. Mental depression leading to Qi stagnation causes accumulation of Body Fluid, which gives rise to Phlegm. The Phlegm brought by the Liver Wind misting the Heart results in mental depression.

Symptoms	Pathogenesis and analysis
Depressive disorder. Mental dejection, dull complexion, murmuring to self with strange behaviours, sticky tongue-coating, rolling pulse	The stagnated Liver-Qi causes mental depression and dull complexion. The Phlegm mists the Heart, the Mind stored in the Heart is disturbed, causing a dull complexion, murmuring and strange behaviours
Epilepsy. Falling down in a fit, loss of consciousness, foam on the lips, Phlegm gurgling in throat, screams with eyes staring upward, convulsions. After a while, consciousness returns. Sticky tongue-coating, rolling pulse	The Liver Wind brings the Phlegm up to mist the Heart, causing falling down in a fit, loss of consciousness, foam on the lips, Phlegm gurgling in the throat. The Liver dominates the tendons, the Liver Wind causes convulsions with eyes staring upward. The Liver-Qi is perverse upward, bringing the Phlegm up to throat and causing screams like a pig or sheep. The excessive Phlegm inside causes a sticky tongue-coating and rolling pulse
Phlegm syncope. Dark complexion, fullness in epigastric region, nausea, cloudiness of consciousness, slurred speech, or even unconsciousness, Phlegm gurgling in throat, white sticky tongue coating, rolling pulse	Invasion of Damp to the Middle Burner causes the failure of ascending of clear Yang and descending of turbid Qi, causing a dark complexion. The abnormal rising of Stomach-Qi causes fullness in the epigastric region and nausea. The accumulation of Damp forms the Phlegm that is brought up to the throat, so gurgling in the throat. The Mind is disturbed by the Phlegm, causing cloudiness of consciousness, slurred speech, or even unconsciousness

Phlegm Fire disturbing the Heart

Pathogenesis and analysis: Coma, delirium, mania plus symptoms of Phlegm Fire.

Emotional disturbance leading to Qi stagnation, which is transformed into Fire condenses the Body Fluid into Phlegm. Or invasion of Damp Heat accumulates into Phlegm Fire. Or invasion of Heat condenses the Body Fluid into Phlegm. The Phlegm Fire disturbs the Mind, causing coma, delirium, or mania with violent behaviours.

Symptoms	Pathogenesis and analysis
In the febrile disease, the manifestations are fever, red face, coarse breathing, constipation, yellow urine, yellow sputum, gurgling sputum in throat, fullness in the chest, or coma, delirium, yellow sticky tongue-coating, rolling rapid pulse	In the febrile disease, the internal Heat is excessive, causing fever, red face, coarse breathing, constipation, and yellow urine. The Heat condenses the Body Fluid into Phlegm, producing yellow sputum, gurgling sputum in throat, and fullness in chest. The Phlegm Fire disturbs the Mind, presenting as coma and delirium. The Phlegm Fire is excessive, causing yellow sticky tongue-coating and rolling rapid pulse
In the endogenous disease, the manifestations are irritability, sleeplessness, mania with violent behaviours, incoherent speech, laughter and crying, red tongue, yellow sticky tongue-coating, rolling rapid pulse	In the endogenous disease, the Phlegm Fire disturbs the Mind, giving rise to irritability and sleeplessness, even mania with violent behaviours, incoherent speech, and laughing and crying

1.5 Excess Heat of the Small Intestine

This is a syndrome with the manifestations of internal Heat in the Small Intestine caused by the Heart Heat moving down to the Small Intestine.

Symptoms	Pathogenesis	Analysis
Irritability, insomnia, thirst with preference for Cold drinks, ulcers of the tongue, or dark yellow urine with painful urination, bloody urine, red tongue, yellow coating, rapid pulse	The Heart Heat moves down to the Small Intestine. Dark yellow urine with painful urination, symptoms of Heart Fire	The Heart Heat moves down to the Small Intestine causing dark yellow urine with painful urination. The Heat injures vessels, causing bloody urine. The Heart Fire disturbs the Mind, causing irritability. The Heat consumes Body Fluid, causing thirst with a preference for Cold drinks. The Heart Fire flares up, causing ulcers of the tongue. The internal Heat causes a red tongue with a yellow coating, and a rapid pulse.

2. SYNDROMES OF THE LUNGS AND LARGE INTESTINE

The Lungs are situated in the thorax, with the Lung Meridian connected with the Large Intestine, with which it is internally–externally related. The Lungs dominate Qi, control respiration, dominate dispersing, skin and hair, dominate descending and regulate the passage of Water.

The Large Intestine receives the waste material sent down from the Small Intestine, absorbs its fluid content, and forms the remainder into faeces to be excreted.

Diseases of the Lung

Pathological changes:

1. Disturbance of respiration.

2. Disorders of Water distribution.

3. Disorders of the defensive function.

4. Disorders of dispersing and descending.

Symptoms: Cough, asthmatic breathing, cough with sputum, distention and pain in chest, obstruction of nose, itching of throat, hoarseness, oedema.

Deficiency syndromes: Deficiency of Lung-Qi, deficiency of Lung Yin.

Excess syndromes: Invasion of the Lungs by Wind Cold, invasion of the Lungs by Wind Heat, invasion of the Lungs by dryness, excessive Heat in the Lungs, retention of Phlegm Heat in the Lungs, invasion of the Lungs by Cold.

Diseases of the Large Intestine

Pathological changes: Disorders of transforming and transporting waste.

Symptoms: Constipation, diarrhoea, abdominal pain, abdominal distention, borborygmus, intestinal flatus from anus, tenesmus.

Deficiency syndromes: Consumption of the fluid of Large Intestine.

Excess syndromes: Damp Heat in the Large Intestine, prolonged diarrhoea due to deficiency of the Large Intestine.

2.1 Invasion of the Lungs by Wind Cold, invasion of the Lungs by Wind Heat

Invasion of the Lungs by Wind Cold: It is a syndrome with the manifestation of dysfunction of the Lungs in dispersing due to invasion of Wind Cold.

Invasion of the Lungs by Wind Heat: It is a syndrome with the manifestation of disorders of defensive Qi due to invasion of the Lungs by Wind Heat.

These two syndromes have the following symptoms in common: cough with sputum, nasal obstruction, nasal discharge, aversion to cold, fever, headache, aching all over the body, superficial pulse.

Invasion of the Lungs by Wind Cold

Symptoms: Cough with thin sputum, aversion to cold with mild fever, nasal obstruction, running nose, no sweating, thin white tongue-coating, superficial tense pulse.

Pathogenesis: Invasion of Wind Cold causes the failure of the Lungs in carrying out their dispersing function.

Analysis: Cough, clear thin white sputum plus exterior Wind Cold syndrome.

Invasion of Wind Cold causes the failure of the Lungs in descending, causing a cough with thin sputum. The failure of Lung-Qi in dispersing causes nasal obstruction and a running nose. The obstruction of defensive Qi causes an aversion to cold. The antipathogenic Qi fights with the pathogenic factors, causing fever. The skin pores are closed by cold, resulting in no sweating. The superficial pulse indicates the exterior, and tense pulse indicates the Cold.

Invasion of the Lungs by Wind Heat

Symptoms: Cough with yellow thick sputum, fever with mild aversion to cold, nasal obstruction with thick discharge, slight thirst, sore throat, red tip of the tongue, thin yellow coating, superficial rapid pulse.

Pathogenesis: Invasion of Wind Heat causes disorders of defensive Qi.

Analysis: Cough with thick yellow sputum plus exterior Wind Heat syndrome.

The invasion of Wind Heat causes the failure of the Lungs in descending, resulting in a cough. Wind Heat is a Yang pathogenic factor that consumes the Body Fluid, leading to yellow thick sputum. The failure of the Lungs in dispersing causes the nasal obstruction, and the Body Fluid being consumed by the Wind Heat, leads to the thick yellow nasal discharge. The obstruction of defensive Qi causes an aversion to the Cold. The Wind Heat disturbs upward and injures the Body Fluid, causing thirst and a sore throat. The superficial pulse indicates the exterior and rapid pulse indicates the Heat.

2.2 Deficiency of Lung Yin, invasion of the Lungs by dryness, deficiency of Lung-Qi

Deficiency of Lung Yin: This is a syndrome with the manifestation of deficiency Heat due to the deficiency of the Yin of the Lungs.

Invasion of the Lungs by dryness: This is a syndrome with the manifestation of injury of the Body Fluid of the Lungs due to the invasion of dryness.

These two syndromes have the following symptoms in common: unproductive cough or cough with sticky sputum that is difficult to spit out, or bloody sputum, dry throat.

Deficiency of Lung-Qi: This is a syndrome with the manifestation of disorders of defensive Qi due to the deficiency of Lung-Qi.

Deficiency of Lung Yin

Symptoms: Emaciation, hot sensation in the Five Centres, afternoon fever, night sweating, flushed cheeks, hoarseness, red tongue without moisture, thready rapid pulse.

Pathogenesis and analysis: The dryness injures the Yin of the Lungs, or sweating consumes the Body Fluid, or a prolonged cough damages the Yin of the Lungs, causing the deficiency Heat and abnormal ascending of Lung-Qi, and leading to a cough.

The Yin fluid is deficient, the body lacks nourishment, causing emaciation. Yin deficiency fails to control Yang and deficiency Heat is produced causing a hot sensation in the Five Centres and afternoon fever. Heat disturbs the Ying-nutrient system, causing night sweating. The deficiency Fire flares up, causing flushed cheeks. The throat is not moistened by Yin and Body Fluid, leading to hoarseness. The internal Heat is produced by Yin deficiency, causing a red tongue without moisture and a thready rapid pulse.

Invasion of the Lungs by dryness

Symptoms: Dry mouth, lips, nose and throat, fever, slight aversion to cold, or chest pain with haemoptysis, thin and dry tongue-coating, rapid pulse.

Pathogenesis and analysis: Cough with little sputum plus exterior syndrome.

The dryness includes warm dryness and cool dryness, warm dryness usually occurring in early autumn and cool dryness in late autumn. The dryness damages the Body Fluid in the Lungs, which then fail to dominate descending, causing a cough with thick sticky sputum and a dry mouth, lips, nose and throat.

The Lung-Qi is defensive. The invasion of dryness causes fever and an aversion to cold because the defensive Qi is damaged. The cool dryness is associated with the tendency of Cold so its manifestation is similar to Wind Cold, while the warm dryness is associated with the tendency of Heat, so its manifestation is similar to Wind Heat. The dryness transformed into Fire that damages the vessels of the Lungs results in chest pain and haemoptysis. The dryness injuring the Body Fluid of the Lungs results in a dry tongue-coating. In most cases, the pulse is rapid when the dryness injures the Lungs.

Deficiency of Lung-Qi

Symptoms: A low-pitched cough which becomes worse on exertion, clear thin sputum, shortness of breath, spontaneous sweating, aversion to Wind, listlessness, pale complexion, pale tongue with a white coating, and a weak pulse.

Pathogenesis and analysis: Cough with clear thin sputum plus symptoms of Qi deficiency.

The prolonged cough consumes the Qi of the Lungs. The Spleen deficiency fails to produce enough Qi and Blood, so the Lungs lack nourishment. The cough is in a low voice because the Lung-Qi is deficient.

The Qi of the Lungs is deficient, the respiration is weak, leading to shortness of breath and a cough in a low voice. The movement consumes Qi, and thus the cough becomes worse. Water is not distributed well since the Lung-Qi is deficient so it is retained in the Lungs causing thin sputum. The deficiency of Lung-Qi causes the low voice, and the defence is weak, causing spontaneous sweating and aversion to Wind. Tiredness, pale complexion and tongue and weak pulse are the signs of Qi deficiency.

2.3 Invasion of the Lungs by Cold, excessive Heat in the Lungs, obstruction of Phlegm Damp in the Lungs

Invasion of the Lungs by Cold: This is a syndrome with the manifestation of the Lungs invaded by the pathogenic Cold.

Excessive Heat in the Lungs: This is a syndrome with the manifestation of failure of Lungs in descending due to excessive Heat in the Lungs.

Obstruction of Phlegm Damp in the Lungs: This is a syndrome with the manifestation of Phlegm Heat obstructing in the Lungs.

Invasion of the Lungs by Cold

Symptoms: Cough, asthmatic breathing, white thin sputum, cold limbs, pale tongue, white coating, slow pulse.

Pathogenesis: Pathogenic Cold invades the Lungs.

Analysis: Sudden onset of cough and asthma plus signs of Cold.

Invasion of Cold obstructs Yang Qi and causes the Qi of the Lung to rise, leading to a cough and asthmatic breathing. Cold is a Yin pathogenic factor, causing thin sputum of a white colour. Yang Qi is not distributed, leading to cold limbs. Pathogenic Cold is characterized by contraction, Qi and Blood circulation stagnates, leading to a pale tongue with a white coating and a slow pulse.

Excessive Heat in the Lungs

Symptoms: Fever, thirst, cough, asthmatic breathing, flaring of nares, chest pain, sore throat, yellow scanty urine, constipation, red tongue, yellow coating, rapid pulse.

Pathogenesis: Pathogenic Wind Heat invades the Lungs or pathogenic Cold is transformed into Heat, which accumulates in the Lungs.

Analysis: Cough, asthmatic breathing, sore throat plus interior Excess Heat syndrome.

Pathogenic Heat accumulates in the Lungs, making the Qi of the Lungs rise, causing a cough. The Body Fluid is condensed into Phlegm, therefore causing thick yellow sputum. The Lungs lose their function of descending, therefore causing asthmatic breathing. The internal Heat is excessive, leading to fever and thirst. Body Fluid is consumed by the internal Heat, leading to constipation and yellow scanty urine. A red tongue with a yellow coating and a rapid pulse are the signs of internal Heat syndrome.

Obstruction of Phlegm Damp in the Lungs

Symptoms: Cough with profuse white sputum which is easily spat out, fullness in the chest, even asthmatic breathing with sputum gurgling in the throat, a pale tongue with a white sticky coating, a rolling pulse.

Pathogenesis: Caused by Spleen-Qi deficiency or damage of Lungs due to prolonged cough or invasion of Cold Damp. Seen in acute and chronic diseases, especially chronic diseases.

In acute diseases, the invasion of Cold Damp to the Lungs causes its failure in distributing the Body Fluid and the retention of water forms sputum. In chronic diseases, the Spleen-Qi deficiency makes the distribution of Water disordered and the retention of water forms sputum that disturbs the Lungs; while in the case of damage to the Lungs due to prolonged cough, the distribution of Water is weakened and the accumulation of Damp forms sputum blocking the Lungs.

Analysis: Cough with profuse white sticky sputum which is easily spat out.

Phlegm Damp blocks the Lungs, making the Lung-Qi rise, causing a cough with profuse sputum, which is white and sticky and easily spat out. Phlegm Damp obstructs the Qi passage, obstructing the Lung-Qi, causing fullness in the chest, even asthmatic breathing. A pale tongue with a white sticky coating, and rolling pulse are the signs of Phlegm Damp.

Differentiation

	Symptoms in common	Distinguishing symptoms
Invasion of the Lungs by Wind Cold	Cough with thin white sputum	In addition to an aversion to cold and fever, which are the symptoms of exterior syndrome, the cough is relatively mild and the duration of disease is short. The pathological condition is of the exterior and interior as both are diseased
Invasion of the Lungs by Cold		Asthmatic breathing, cold limbs, no fever, serious cough, long duration of disease, belonging to the interior syndrome

2.4 Damp Heat in the Large Intestine, prolonged diarrhoea due to deficiency of the Large Intestine, consumption of the fluid of the Large Intestine

Damp Heat in the Large Intestine: Invasion of Damp Heat causes the Large Intestine to become disordered in sending the wastes down to be discharged, mainly manifesting as diarrhoea with tenesmus.

Prolonged diarrhoea due to deficiency of the Large Intestine: Manifestations of deficiency of Yang Qi of Large Intestine.

The last two mentioned have the following symptoms in common: abdominal pain, diarrhoea.

Consumption of the fluid of the Large Intestine: Body Fluid of the Large Intestine is deficient, failing to transport the wastes, causing dry stools.

Damp Heat in the Large Intestine

Symptoms: Abdominal pain, diarrhoea with purulent and bloody stools, tenesmus, or spouting diarrhoea with stinking stools, accompanied by a hot sensation in the anus, fever, thist, scanty yellow urine, a red tongue with a yellow sticky coating, and a rolling rapid pulse.

Pathogenesis: In summer and autumn, the invasion of Summer Heat and Damp to the intestines or the intake of contaminated food causes the obstruction of the intestines by Damp Heat turbidity.

Analysis: Dysentery with bloody purulent stools, diarrhoea, abdominal pain, tenesmus plus symptoms of Damp Heat.

The invasion of Damp causes Qi obstruction, causing abdominal pain. The intestinal collaterals are damaged by Heat, forming the bloody, purulent stools. The Heat steams in the intestines, leading to intestinal hyperperistalsis, thus causing abdominal pain. The intestinal obstruction by Damp results in irregular discharge of faeces, and therefore tenesmus. When the Large Intestine is affected by Damp Heat, the Body Fluid is forced downwards, resulting in frequent bowel movements with yellow watery stools. The Heat in the intestines produces a hot sensation in the anus. The Water goes to the stools, so there is scanty yellow urine. The Heat consumes Body Fluid, giving rise to thirst. The red tongue, yellow coating, and rolling rapid pulse are the signs of Damp Heat.

Prolonged diarrhoea due to deficiency of the Large Intestine

Symptoms: Borborygmus, loose stools or incontinence, proctoptosis, dull pain in abdomen that is better with warmth and pressure, pale tongue with white wet coating, deep weak pulse.

Pathogenesis: Constitutional Yang deficiency and the damage of Yang Qi from overconsumption of raw and Cold food, or prolonged diseases, or long-term diarrhoea.

Analysis: Prolonged diarrhoea or incontinence of stools plus symptoms of deficiency Cold.

The weakness of Yang Qi caused by long-term diarrhoea results in the failure of Large Intestine to control, leading to incontinence of stools and proctoptosis. The internal Cold from Yang deficiency with Yin excess causes Cold stagnation and Qi obstruction, causing a dull pain in the abdomen, which is better on warmth and pressure. A pale tongue with a white wet coating and deep weak pulse are the signs of Deficiency Cold syndrome.

Consumption of the fluid of Large Intestine

Symptoms: Constipation with dry stools that are difficult to discharge, dry mouth or bad smell from the mouth, dizziness, red tongue with yellow dry coating, thready hesitant pulse.

Pathogenesis: In addition to constitutional Yin deficiency and Yin Blood deficiency due to old age, diarrhoea and vomiting, prolonged disease, late stage of a febrile disease, a loss of blood and profuse bleeding after delivery can all cause consumption of Yin fluid, manifesting as constipation with dry stools because the Large Intestine is poorly moistened.

Analysis: Constipation with dry stools plus symptoms of Body Fluid deficiency.

The Large Intestine lacks moisture due to Body Fluid deficiency, causing dry stools that are difficult to discharge. The mouth and throat are not moistened because of the consumption of Yin fluid, leading to a dry mouth and throat. The dry stools stay in the Large Intestine for a long time, causing turbid Qi to rise, and resulting in foul breath and dizziness. The red tongue without moisture is from Yin consumption and Yang excess. The thready hesitant pulse is from the Body Fluid consumption and poor filling up of vessels.

3. SYNDROMES OF THE SPLEEN AND STOMACH

The Spleen and Stomach are located in the Middle Burner, and their meridians are externally–internally related to each other. The former, with its Qi that ascends, dominates transportation and transformation of food and Water, while the latter, with its Qi that descends, receives food for digestion. In combination with each other, they function to absorb and distribute nutrients. Being the production source of Qi and Blood, the Spleen and Stomach are regarded as the acquired foundation of the human body. And the Spleen also controls Blood and dominates the four limbs and muscles.

Diseases of the Spleen

Pathological changes:

1. The Spleen dominating the transportation and transformation fails, Qi and Blood production is deficient, Phlegm is produced, and Damp formed.

2. The Spleen controlling Blood becomes disordered, bleeding appears.

3. The Spleen-Qi sinks, the clean Yang stops going upward.

Symptoms: Abdominal distention and pain, poor appetite, loose stools, oedema, heaviness of limbs, emaciation, various kinds of bleeding.

Deficiency syndromes: Deficiency of Spleen-Qi, deficiency of Spleen Yang, sinking of Qi of Middle Burner, Spleen failing to control Blood.

Excess syndromes: Retention of Damp Heat in Spleen, Cold Damp affecting Spleen.

Diseases of the Stomach

Pathological changes:

1. Disorders in receiving and digesting food.

2. The Stomach-Qi going upward abnormally.

Symptoms: Epigastric distention and pain, eating less, eating a lot but still hungry, belching, hiccups, nausea, and vomiting.

Deficiency syndromes: Deficiency of Stomach Yin.

Excess syndromes: Retention of food in Stomach, Stomach Cold, Stomach Heat.

3.1 Deficiency of Spleen-Qi, deficiency of Spleen Yang

Deficiency of Spleen-Qi: Manifestations of Spleen failing to transport and transform food and Water.

Deficiency of Spleen Yang: Manifestations of internal Cold resulting from the failure of Spleen Yang to warm the interior.

These syndromes have the following symptoms in common: poor appetite, abdominal distention (especially after eating), loose stools, shortness of breath, reduced speech, tiredness, sallow or pale complexion, pale tongue with white coating, pulse a bit weak and slow.

Deficiency of Spleen-Qi

Symptoms: Emaciation, oedema.

Pathogenesis and analysis: Poor appetite, abdominal distention, loose stools plus symptoms of Qi deficiency.

After eating, the Spleen-Qi is easily weakened, so abdominal distention gets worse. When the Spleen-Qi is weak, the Stomach-Qi will be weak too, and consequently the digesting function is weak, causing one to eat less. Water is not well transported by the Spleen, and goes to the Large Intestine, causing loose stools. The poor transportation and transformation of the Spleen leads to poor nourishment of the limbs, causing tiredness, shortness of breath, and inactive talking. The Spleen is deficient in producing Qi and Blood, causing a sallow or pale complexion. A pale tongue with white coating is the sign of Spleen-Qi deficiency, and Qi and Blood deficiency owing to Spleen failure or Damp invasion to the skin results in emaciation and oedema.

Deficiency of Spleen Yang

Symptoms: Abdominal pain which is alleviated by warmth and pressure, cold limbs, heaviness of limbs, oedema all over the body, scanty urine, profuse thin leucorrhoea, pale flabby tongue with white wet coating, deep slow weak pulse.

Pathogenesis and analysis: Symptoms of Spleen-Qi deficiency plus symptoms of deficiency Cold.

This is developed from the Spleen-Qi deficiency, or is due to over-eating Cold and raw food, or an over-dosage of Cold medicine damaging the Spleen Yang or Kidney Yang and causing interior Cold. The Cold contraction and Qi stagnation caused by interior Cold results in abdominal pain that is alleviated by warmth and pressure. The deficient Spleen Yang fails to warm the limbs, leading to cold limbs. The Spleen Yang deficiency causes the retention of water and Qi activity of Bladder disorders, which result in scanty urine. Water stays in the skin, leading to heaviness of limbs and oedema all over the body. The Dai-Belt Vessel is unconsolidated, the Water Damp flows downward, causing profuse thin leucorrhoea. A pale flabby tongue with a white wet coating and deep slow weak pulse are the signs of Yang deficiency with interior Cold Water.

3.2 Sinking of Qi of Middle Burner, Spleen failing to control Blood

Sinking of Qi of Middle Burner: Manifestations of deficiency of Spleen-Qi failing to lift.

Spleen failing to control Blood: Manifestations of Spleen-Qi deficiency symptomized by extravasation of Blood.

Sinking of Qi of Middle Burner

Symptoms: Abdominal distention, especially after eating, frequent desire to discharge stools with a bearing-down sensation in the anus, prolonged diarrhoea, prolapse of rectum, prolapse of uterus, turbid urine like rice water, dizziness, blurred vision, poor appetite, loose stools, shortness of breath, tiredness, inactive talking, pale complexion, pale tongue with white coating, weak and a rather slow pulse.

Pathogenesis: This develops from Spleen-Qi deficiency, or Spleen-Qi damage due to prolonged diarrhoea, overworking, or careless nursing after delivery. The deficient Spleen-Qi gives inadequate nourishment to the internal organs, the Qi of which fails to keep them in the right position, with gastroptosis being the most commonly seen symptom in clinic.

Analysis: Symptoms of Spleen-Qi deficiency plus visceral ptosis.

After eating, the sinking of Qi becomes more serious, and the bearing-down sensation in the abdomen becomes worse. There is a frequent desire to discharge stools with a bearing-down sensation in the anus, prolonged diarrhoea, prolapse of the rectum, and prolapse of the uterus, which are all manifestations of the sinking of the Qi of the Middle Burner. The Spleen deficiency and sinking of Qi cause the nutrient to fail to distribute, thus flowing to the Bladder, creating turbid urine like rice water. The deficiency of the Qi of the Middle Burner causes hypofunction of the whole body, causing a poor appetite, loose stools, shortness of breath, tiredness, inactive talking, and a pale complexion. Clean Yang fails to ascend, causing dizziness and blurred vision. A pale tongue with a white coating, and a weak and a rather slow pulse are signs of Spleen-Qi deficiency.

Spleen failing to control Blood

Symptoms: Sallow or pale complexion, listlessness, shortness of breath, inactive talking, poor appetite, loose stools, bloody stools, bloody urine, haematohidrosis, epistaxis, menorrhagia, uterine functional bleeding, pale tongue, thready forceless pulse.

Pathogenesis: Qi deficiency due to a prolonged disease, or overworking damaging the Spleen-Qi, makes the function of Spleen in controlling Blood become lost, causing bleeding.

Analysis: Symptoms of Spleen-Qi deficiency plus bleeding.

Blood is extravasated to intestines, causing bloody stools; to the Bladder, causing bloody urine; to the subcutaneous region, causing Blood spots on the skin; to the skin pores, causing haematohidrosis. Chong-Thoroughfare and Ren-Conception are not consolidated, causing menorrhagia and uterine functional bleeding. The hypofunction of the Spleen in transportation and transformation leads to a poor appetite and loose stools. Listlessness, shortness of breath, and inactive talking come from a deficiency of Qi of the Middle Burner. Repeated bleeding causes Blood deficiency which results in a sallow or pale complexion. A pale tongue and thready forceless pulse are the signs of Qi deficiency.

Differentiation

	Symptoms in common	Distinguishing symptoms
Deficiency of Spleen-Qi	Poor appetite, abdominal distention, especially after eating, loose stools, tiredness, inactive talking, sallow complexion	Emaciation or oedema. Pale tongue with white coating. Weak retarded pulse
Deficiency of Spleen Yang		Abdominal pain which is better on warmth and pressure, cold limbs, scanty urine, heaviness of limbs, oedema, white thin leucorrhoea. Pale flabby tongue, white wet coating. Deep slow weak pulse
Sinking of Qi of Middle Burner		Abdominal distention, frequent desire to discharge stools with a bearing-down sensation in the anus, prolonged diarrhoea, prolapse of rectum, prolapse of uterus, turbid urine like rice water. Pale tongue with white coating. Weak pulse
Spleen failing to control Blood		Bloody stools, bloody urine, haematohidrosis, epistaxis, gum bleeding, menorrhagia, uterine functional bleeding. Pale tongue, white coating. Thready weak pulse

3.3 Cold Damp affecting Spleen, retention of Damp Heat in Spleen

Cold Damp affecting Spleen: Manifestations of Spleen Yang affected by the excessive interior Cold Damp.

Retention of Damp Heat in Spleen: Manifestations of Spleen and Stomach disorders in transportation and transformation and receiving food caused by accumulation of Damp Heat in the Middle Burner.

These syndromes have the following symptoms in common: fullness and distention in epigastrium and abdomen, nausea, poor appetite, loose stools, heaviness of head and body, jaundice with dark yellow skin and sclera, sticky tongue-coating, and a thready soft weak pulse.

Cold Damp affecting Spleen

Symptoms: Fullness and distending pain in epigastrium and abdomen, nausea, lack of taste and absence of thirst, heaviness of head and body, oedema of limbs, scanty urine, jaundice with dark yellow skin and sclera, pale flabby tongue, white sticky coating, thready soft weak and a rather slow pulse.

Pathogenesis: Irregular food intake and over-eating of raw and Cold food cause the retention of Cold Damp in the Middle Burner. Being caught in the rain or living in a Damp place leads to the invasion of Cold Damp to the Middle Burner. Over-eating of fatty food produces Damp turbidity, which obstructs Yang of the Middle Burner.

Analysis: Disturbance of Spleen in transportation and transformation plus symptoms of retention of Cold Damp in the Middle Burner.

Retention of Cold Damp in the Middle Burner causes the disordered transportation and transformation of the Spleen, causing fullness and a distending pain in epigastrium and abdomen. The Damp is characterized by heaviness and turbidity, causing heaviness of the head and body and oedema of the limbs. Damp blocks Qi, and Qi and Blood circulation is stagnated, failing to nourish and moisten the skin, and causing a dark complexion. Cold Damp makes Yang Qi obstructed and blocks the out-flow of bile, causing jaundice. Cold Damp blocks Yang Qi, the failure of which in dissolving Damp causes Water to flow to the skin, causing oedema. The dysfunction of the Qi activity of the Bladder produces scanty urine. A pale tongue with a white sticky coating, and a thready, soft, weak and rather slow pulse are the signs of interior Cold Damp.

Retention of Damp Heat in the Spleen

Symptoms: Fullness in the epigastrium and abdomen, poor appetite, nausea, loose stools with non-smooth discharge, scanty urine, heaviness of limbs, feverish sensation of the body which is not relieved by sweating, jaundice with fresh yellow skin and sclera, itching, red tongue with a yellow sticky coating and a thready soft weak and rapid pulse.

Pathogenesis: Invasion of Damp Heat, over-eating of spicy fatty food, and indulgence in alcohol cause the formation of Damp Heat which accumulates in the Spleen and Stomach.

Analysis: Disturbance of the Spleen in transportation and transformation plus symptoms of retention of Damp Heat in the Middle Burner.

Damp Heat accumulates in the Spleen and Stomach and the transportation and transformation function of the Spleen and the food receiving function of the Stomach become disordered, leading to fullness in the epigastrium and abdomen, a poor appetite, and nausea. Damp is characterized by heaviness, and the Spleen is affected by Damp, causing heaviness of limbs. Damp Heat retention in the Spleen forces Water into the Large Intestine, causing loose stools with irregular discharge and scanty urine. Damp Heat steams the interior, affecting the Liver and Gallbladder, and the bile goes abnormally to the skin, causing jaundice with bright yellow skin and sclera and itching. Damp obstruction with Heat accumulation produces a feverish sensation in the body which isn't relieved by sweating. A red tongue with a yellow sticky coating, thready soft weak and rapid pulse are signs of the accumulation of Damp Heat in the interior.

3.4 Deficiency of Stomach Yin, Stomach Heat

Deficiency of Stomach Yin: Manifestations of the Stomach being poorly moistened due to Stomach Yin deficiency and failure of the Stomach-Qi to descend.

Stomach Heat: Manifestations of excess Heat in the Stomach making its Qi fail to descend.

These syndromes have the following symptoms in common: burning pain in the epigastrium, dry mouth, thirst, constipation, yellow scanty urine, and a rapid pulse.

Deficiency of Stomach Yin

Symptoms: Dull pain and fullness in the epigastrium, hunger but without a desire to eat, dry mouth and throat, constipation with dry stools, nausea, hiccups, red tongue without moisture, and a thready rapid pulse.

Pathogenesis: The Stomach Yin is damaged in the late stage of febrile disease. Emotional depression causes Qi stagnation, which transforms into Fire, damaging the Stomach Yin. Severe vomiting consumes the Body Fluid. Over-eating spicy food or over-dosage of medicine that is of a warm and dry nature consumes the Stomach Yin.

Analysis: Symptoms of Stomach-Qi ascending plus symptoms of Stomach Yin deficiency.

Internal Heat is produced by Stomach Yin deficiency and the Heat stagnates in the Stomach, causing a dull pain and fullness in the epigastrium and hunger but without a desire to eat. The Stomach Yin is deficient, so the mouth and throat lack moisture, a dry mouth and throat appear, while the Large Intestine is poorly moistened, causing constipation with dry stools. The Stomach is not moistened by Stomach Yin, its Qi is not harmonized, going upward instead of going down normally, also epigastric fullness, nausea and hiccups appear. A red tongue without moisture and a thready rapid pulse are the signs of internal Heat due to Yin deficiency.

Stomach Heat

Symptoms: A burning pain in the epigastrium, which is worse on pressure, acid regurgitation, thirst with a desire to drink Cold water, eating a lot but still feeling hungry, foul breath, swelling and painful gums, bleeding gums, constipation, yellow scanty urine, red tongue with a yellow coating, and a rolling rapid pulse.

Pathogenesis: Over-eating spicy food produces Fire. Emotional depression causes Qi stagnation which affects the Stomach. Invasion of pathogenic Heat gives rise to excessive Stomach Fire.

Analysis: Symptoms of epigastric burning pain plus symptoms of excessive internal Fire.

A burning pain in the epigastrium is caused by Fire in the Stomach blocking its Qi and Blood. The Liver Fire overacts on the Stomach, causing acid regurgitation. The Stomach Fire burns Body Fluids, so there is thirst with a desire to drink Cold Water. The hyperfunction that brought Fire causes one to eat a lot but still feel hungry. The collateral of the Stomach distributes to the gums, and the Stomach Fire goes to the gums, causing swelling and painful and bleeding gums. The turbid Qi of the Stomach ascends, causing foul breath. Fire consumes Body Fluid, causing constipation and yellow scanty urine. A red tongue with a yellow coating, and a rolling rapid pulse are the signs of Heat syndrome.

3.5 Stomach Cold

This refers to those manifestations of Cold pain in the epigastrium caused by an invasion of Cold.

Symptoms: Cold pain in epigastrium, which is made worse by exposure to Cold and better by warmth, no thirst, pale or blue complexion, cold limbs, pale tongue, white wet coating, wiry or deep tight pulse.

Pathogenesis: Over-eating raw or Cold food and invasion of Cold to epigastrium leads to retention of Cold in the Stomach.

Analysis: Epigastric Cold pain plus symptoms of excess Cold.

Pathogenic Cold blocking the Stomach makes the Stomach-Qi stagnate, causing Cold pain. Pathogenic Cold damages Yang, without which Water fluid can't be dissolved, resulting in a lack of thirst. Yang Qi fails to move outwards because of Cold obstruction, causing a pale or blue complexion and cold limbs. A pale tongue with a white wet coating, wiry or deep tight pulse are the signs of excessive Yin Cold blocking the Qi circulation.

3.6 Retention of food in Stomach

This refers to those manifestations of fullness and distending pain in the epigastrium and abdomen, vomiting and diarrhoea that are due to food retention in the Stomach.

Symptoms: Fullness, distention and possibly pain in the epigastrium, belching, acid regurgitation, vomiting, borborygmus with abdominal pain, diarrhoea with stinking stools, thick sticky tongue-coating, rolling or deep forceful pulse.

Pathogenesis: A dysfunction of the Spleen in transportation and transformation is caused by voracious eating or a constitutional deficiency of the Spleen and Stomach.

Analysis: Epigastric distending pain plus vomiting.

Retention of food makes the Stomach-Qi fail to descend, carry fullness and distention or even pain in the epigastrium. The obstructed Stomach-Qi brings the undigested food upward, causing belching, acid regurgitation and vomiting. Fullness and distending pain are relieved after vomiting because the Stomach-Qi thus becomes unobstructed. The Qi movement of the Large Intestine is blocked by food retention, causing borborygmus, abdominal pain, and diarrhoea with stinking stools. The turbid Stomach-Qi steams upward, causing a thick sticky tongue-coating. The rolling and deep forceful pulse is the sign of food retention.

Differentiation

	Symptoms
Stomach Cold	Cold pain, which is made worse by exposure to Cold and better by warmth and pressure. No thirst. Pain relieved by warm food. Vomiting of clear Water. Loose stools. Intestinal watery sound, cold limbs, listlessness. Pale tongue, white wet coating. Slow or wiry tight pulse
Stomach Heat	Burning pain. Thirst with desire to drink Cold Water, foul breath. Eating a lot but still feeling hungry, or vomiting after eating. Acid regurgitation. Loose stools, yellow urine. Painful, swelling and bleeding gums. Red tongue with a yellow coating. Rolling rapid pulse
Deficiency of Stomach Yin	Dull pain. Dry mouth and throat with desire to drink. Hungry but without a desire to eat. Nausea, hiccups. Constipation. Epigastric fullness, emaciation. Red tongue with little coating. Thready rapid pulse
Retention of food in Stomach	Distending pain. Foul breath. Intolerance of food smells. Belching, acid regurgitation, vomiting. Flatulence, loose stools, diarrhoea with stinking stools or constipation. Thick sticky coating. Rolling pulse

4. SYNDROMES OF THE LIVER AND GALLBLADDER

The Liver is located in the right hypochondrium. Its meridian connects with the Gallbladder, with which it is externally–internally related. The Liver stores Blood, maintains the free flow of Qi, controls the tendons with its manifestation in nails, and opens into the eye. The Gallbladder stores bile and continuously excretes this into the intestines in order to aid digestion and relating to mental activities.

Diseases of the Liver

Pathological changes:

1. Disorders in maintaining free flow of Qi.
2. Failure to control Blood.
3. Deficiency of Yin Blood depriving tendons of nourishment.
4. Stirring up Wind and transforming into Fire.

Symptoms: Mental depression, irritability, distending pain in hypochondrium and lower abdomen, dizziness, tremor, convulsion, diseases of the eyes, menstruation disorders, pain of the external genitalia.

Deficiency syndromes: Blood deficiency of the Liver, Yin deficiency of the Liver.

Excess syndromes: Qi stagnation of the Liver, flare-up of the Liver Fire, retention of Cold in the Liver Meridian, Damp Heat in the Liver and Gallbladder.

Ben-deficiency Biao-excess syndromes: Rising of the Liver Yang.

Stirring of the Liver Wind syndromes: Liver Yang turning into Wind, extreme Heat producing Wind, Yin deficiency stirring Wind, Blood deficiency producing Wind.

Diseases of the Gallbladder

Pathological changes:

1. Bile extravasated to the skin.
2. Inability to make decisions.

Symptoms: Bitter taste in mouth, jaundice, timidity, hesitation, insomnia.

Excess syndromes: Qi stagnation of the Gallbladder with disturbance of Phlegm, Damp Heat in the Liver and Gallbladder.

4.1 Blood deficiency of the Liver, Yin deficiency of the Liver

Blood deficiency of the Liver: Manifestations of those tissues and organs, related to the Liver, deprived of nutrients.

Yin deficiency of the Liver: Manifestations of disturbance by deficiency Heat resulting from Liver Yin deficiency that fails to control Yang.

These two syndromes have the following symptoms in common: dizziness and vertigo, tinnitus, blurred vision.

Blood deficiency of the Liver

Symptoms: Dizziness and vertigo, tinnitus, pallor, pale nails, blurring of vision, night blindness, numbness of the limbs, spasms of the tendons, tremor, muscular twitching, scanty menstrual flow or amenorrhoea, pale tongue with white coating, thready pulse.

Pathogenesis: Caused by deficiency of Spleen and Stomach producing inadequate Qi and Blood, loss of Blood, prolonged disease, or deficiency of Blood.

Analysis: Symptoms of poor nourishment of muscles, tendons, eyes and nails, plus symptoms of Blood deficiency.

Blood deficiency of the Liver gives poor blood supply to the head and face, causing dizziness and vertigo, tinnitus, and pallor. The nails are deprived of nourishment, and become fragile. The eyes are poorly nourished, causing blurring of vision and night blindness. The muscles and tendons lack nourishment, leading to numbness of the limbs and spasms of the tendons. Tremor and muscular twitching are caused by deficiency Wind stirring. Chong and Ren Meridians are deficient due to the Blood deficiency of the Liver, leading to scanty menstrual flow or amenorrhoea. A pale tongue with a white coating, and thready pulse are the signs of Blood deficiency.

Yin deficiency of the Liver

Symptoms: Dizziness, tinnitus like a cicada ringing, dry sensation in the eyes, a dull burning pain in the hypochondrium, declined vision, flushed cheeks, hot sensation in the Five Centres, afternoon fever, night sweating, dry mouth and throat, involuntary movement of limbs, a red tongue without moisture, and a wiry thready rapid pulse.

Pathogenesis: Qi stagnation due to mental depression transforms into Fire, which consumes the Liver Yin. In the late stage of febrile disease, the Liver Yin is damaged. The Kidney Yin deficiency fails to moisten the Liver Wood, causing Liver Yin deficiency.

Analysis: Symptoms of poor nourishment of muscles, tendons, head and eyes plus symptoms of Yin deficiency with internal Heat.

The Liver Yin deficiency deprives the head and eyes of nourishment, causing dizziness, tinnitus, and a dry sensation in the eyes. The deficiency causes Fire to flare up, causing flushed cheeks. The Fire deficiency burns the Liver collaterals, causing a burning pain in the hypochondriac. The internal Heat due to Yin deficiency disturbs the Ying-nutrient system, causing a hot sensation in the Five Centres, afternoon fever, and night sweating. The dry sensation in the mouth and throat is due to Yin deficiency causing a lack of moisture to moisten the mouth and throat. The muscles and tendons are poorly nourished by the Liver Yin deficiency, resulting in involuntary movement of limbs. A wiry thready rapid pulse is the sign of the internal Heat due to Liver Yin deficiency.

4.2 Qi stagnation of the Liver, retention of Cold in the Liver Meridian

Qi stagnation of the Liver: Manifestations of disorders of the Liver in maintaining the free flow of Qi.

Retention of Cold in the Liver Meridian: Manifestations of Cold pain along the distribution of the Liver Meridian where the pathogenic Cold stagnates.

Qi stagnation of the Liver

Symptoms: Mental depression, distending pain and mass in the hypochondrium and lower abdomen, sighing, the sensation of a foreign body in the throat, goitre, scrofula, swelling of breasts, dysmenorrhoea, irregular menstruation, amenorrhoea, thin white tongue-coating, wiry or hesitant pulse. The pathological changes are relieved or aggravated by the emotional factors.

Pathogenesis: Caused by emotional depression or mental irritation, there is an invasion of pathogens which obstruct the Liver Meridian, resulting in failure of the Liver to maintain the free flow of Qi.

Analysis: Mental depression, distending pain in hypochondrium and abdomen, irregular menstruation.

The Liver-Qi is stagnated, causing mental depression, and a distending pain and mass in the hypochondrium, lower abdomen and breasts. The Liver is disordered in maintaining the free flow of Qi, causing mental depression. Phlegm is produced when Qi is stagnated and brought up to the throat, causing the sensation of a foreign body in the throat. Phlegm accumulates in the neck region, causing goitre and scrofula. Qi stagnation causes Blood stasis, Chong and Ren are not harmonious, causing dysmenorrhoea, irregular menstruation, or even amenorrhoea. The prolonged Qi stagnation and Blood stasis produces hypochondriac mass.

Retention of Cold in the Liver meridian

Symptoms: Cold pain in the lower abdomen with a bearing-down and contracted sensation in the testes, aggravated by Cold and alleviated by warmth, a pale tongue with a white slippery coating, deep wiry slow pulse.

Pathogenesis: Caused by invasion of Cold stagnating in the Liver Meridian.

Analysis: Cold pain with a bearing-down sensation in the lower abdomen and external genitalia plus symptoms of interior Excess Cold syndrome.

The Liver Meridian of Foot Jueyin distributes to the lower abdomen and curves around the external genitalia. The invasion of the Liver Meridian by pathogenic Cold blocks its Yang Qi and Qi and Blood circulation is obstructed, causing a Cold pain in the lower abdomen with a bearing-down sensation in the testes. Cold is characterized by contraction, so a bearing-down and contracted sensation in the testes. Cold makes Qi and Blood stagnate while warmth makes them circulate, and thus the pain is aggravated by Cold and alleviated by warmth. Yin Cold is excessive in the interior, causing a pale tongue with a white slippery coating. A deep pulse indicates an interior syndrome, a wiry one means Liver disease, and a slow one relates to a Yin Cold syndrome.

4.3 Flare-up of Liver Fire, rising of the Liver Yang

Flare-up of the Liver Fire: Manifestations of disorders caused by Liver Fire and stagnated Qi.

Rising of the Liver Yang: Manifestations of upward-excess and downward-deficiency due to Liver Yang disturbing the upper part caused by Yin deficiency of the Liver and the Kidney.

These two syndromes have the following symptoms in common: dizziness and vertigo, tinnitus, headache with distending sensation in the head and eyes, a flushed face, red eyes, irritability, palpitations, a poor memory, and insomnia with dream-disturbed sleep.

Flare-up of Liver Fire

Symptoms: Dizziness, a distending pain in the head, redness, swelling and pain of the eyes, a bitter taste and dryness in the mouth, irritability, insomnia or dream-disturbed sleep, a burning pain in the hypochondrium, constipation, scanty yellow urine, tinnitus like the sound of waves, a sudden loss of hearing, swelling and pain in the ears, haematemesis, epistaxis, red tongue with yellow coating, wiry rapid pulse.

Pathogenesis: Caused by the stagnation of Liver-Qi turning into Fire, and an invasion of pathogenic Heat; the Heat of the other Zang organs influence the Liver and Gallbladder Fire, and stagnated Qi is disturbed and rises.

Analysis: Symptoms of excess Fire in the distribution regions of the Liver Meridian, including the head, eyes, ears, and hypochondrium.

The Fire flares upward along the Liver Meridian, causing dizziness, a distending pain in the head, redness, swelling and pain in the eyes. The Liver Heat transmits to the Gallbladder, the Qi of which brings the Heat upward, causing a bitter taste in the mouth. The Heat consumes the Body Fluid, resulting in dryness in the mouth. The Liver loses its function in maintaining the free flow of Qi, causing irritability. The Fire disturbs the Heart, causes mental restlessness and therefore insomnia or dream-disturbed sleep. The Liver Fire causes the obstruction of Qi and Blood, leading to a burning pain in the hypochondrium. Heat consumes Body Fluid, causing constipation and scanty yellow urine. The Gallbladder Meridian enters the ear, the Liver Fire moves to the Gallbladder and rushes upward, causing tinnitus like the sound of waves or even a sudden loss of hearing. Heat steams in the ear, blocking the Ying-nutrient, and forming a swelling pain there. Heat forces the Blood to extravasate, causing haematemesis and epistaxis. The red tongue with a yellow coating and a wiry pulse are the signs of Liver excess Fire.

Rising of the Liver Yang

Symptoms: Dizziness and vertigo, tinnitus, headache with distending sensation in the head and eyes, flushed face and red eyes, irritability, palpitations, poor memory, insomnia with dream-disturbed sleep, soreness and weakness of the lumbus and knees, feeling heaviness in the head and weakness in the legs, a red tongue, wiry or wiry thready pulse.

Pathogenesis: Caused by Yin deficiency of the Liver and Kidney, mental depression, anger and anxiety. Qi stagnation of the Liver turns into Fire, which consumes the Yin Blood in the interior, causing Yang to rise without Yin's control.

Analysis: Upward rising of Liver Yang, downward deficiency of Kidney Yin.

In Yin deficiency of the Liver and Kidney, excessive ascending of the Yang and Qi of the Liver causes dizziness and vertigo, tinnitus, headache with a distending sensation in the head and eyes, and a flushed face and red eyes. The Liver loses its function in maintaining the free flow of Qi, causing irritability. When there is deficiency of Yin leading to the Heart being poorly nourished, the Mind is disturbed, causing palpitations, poor memory, and insomnia with dream-disturbed sleep. The lumbus houses the Kidneys and the knee houses the tendons, and when there is Yin deficiency of the Liver and Kidneys and the tendons lack nourishment, soreness and weakness of the lumbus and knees will appear. Rising of the Liver Yang (upward excess), and Yin deficiency of the Liver and Kidneys (downward deficiency), lead to a feeling of heaviness in the head and weakness in the legs. A red tongue and wiry or wiry thready pulse are the signs of Yin deficiency of the Liver and Kidneys, with rising of Liver Yang.

4.4 Stirring of the Liver Wind syndromes

The occurrence of dizziness and vertigo, convulsion, and tremor, said to be the 'internal Wind' in pathogenesis, relate to an imbalance between Yin and Yang of the Zang Fu organs, especially the Liver, which is referred to as 'stirring of the Liver Wind'.

Liver Yang turning into Wind: Manifestations of internal Wind caused by excessive ascending of Liver Yang.

Extreme Heat producing Wind: Manifestations of internal Wind caused by pathogenic Heat consuming the Body Fluid, resulting in malnutrition of the tendons and muscles.

Yin deficiency stirring Wind: Manifestations of internal Wind caused by deficiency of Yin fluid leading to malnutrition of tendons and muscles.

Blood deficiency producing Wind: Manifestations of internal Wind caused by deficiency of Blood bringing on malnutrition of the tendons and muscles.

Liver Yang turning into Wind

Symptoms: Dizziness and vertigo, shaking of the head or headache, numbness or tremor of the limbs, dysphasia, falling down in a fit with loss of consciousness, deviation of the mouth and eyes, hemiplegia, stiff tongue, red tongue with a white or sticky coating, wiry forceful pulse.

Pathogenesis: With emotional depression, the Qi stagnation turns into Fire consuming Yin. In constitutional Yin deficiency of Liver and Kidneys, the uncontrolled Liver Yang transforms into Wind, presenting a syndrome of Ben-deficiency Biao-excess and upward-excess downward-deficiency.

Analysis: Symptoms of rising of the Liver Yang such as dizziness and vertigo and blurred vision plus signs of stirring Wind all of a sudden, or falling down in a fit with loss of consciousness and hemiplegia.

The Liver Yang transforms into Wind disturbing upward, causing dizziness, vertigo, and shaking of the head. Wind brings Qi and Blood up and blocks the meridians and collaterals of the head, causing a headache. Wind causes spasm of the tendons, producing tremor of the limbs. Wind Yang disturbs the collateral of the Liver Meridian, which connects with the tongue, causing dysphasia.

The Yin deficiency of the Liver and Kidneys causing the malnutrition of tendons and muscles is the reason for the numbness of limbs. Wind in the upper part of the body (up-excess) and Yin deficiency in the lower part of the body (down-deficiency) produce unsteady walking. Wind Yang ascending suddenly followed by disordered Qi and Blood causes Phlegm to be brought up by the Liver Wind thus disturbing the Mind stored in the Heart, and causing falling down in a fit with a loss of consciousness. Wind and Phlegm block the meridians, the Qi of which is obstructed, causing deviation of the mouth and eyes, hemiplegia, and stiff tongue. A red tongue is the sign of Yin deficiency, a white coating indicates that Fire is not yet formed, and the sticky coating shows the Phlegm has been brought up. A wiry forceful pulse shows the presence of the Yin deficiency of the Liver and Kidney with a rising of the Liver Yang.

Extreme Heat producing Wind

Symptoms: High fever, coma, mania, convulsion, neck rigidity, opisthotonus, upward staring of the eyes, clenched jaws, red or deep red tongue, wiry rapid pulse.

Pathogenesis: In the febrile diseases, the pathogenic Heat burns the Liver Meridian.

Analysis: High fever plus stirring Wind.

Excessive Heat causes high fever. The Heat enters the Pericardium, the Mind is disturbed, causing coma and mania. Heat burns the Liver Meridian and consumes the Body Fluid, stirring the Wind, causing convulsions, neck rigidity, opisthotonus, upward staring of the eyes, and clenched jaws. Heat affects the Ying Blood, causing a red or deep red tongue. A wiry rapid pulse is the sign of Fire burning the Liver Meridian.

Yin deficiency stirring Wind

Symptoms: Involuntary movement of the limbs, dizziness and vertigo, tinnitus, afternoon fever, flushed cheeks, dry mouth and throat, emaciation, red tongue without moisture, thready rapid pulse.

Pathogenesis: Caused by the malnutrition of tendons and muscles resulting from consumption of Yin fluid in the late stage of a febrile disease, or deficiency of Body Fluid due to a prolonged disease.

Analysis: Symptoms of stirring Wind such as involuntary movement of limbs and dizziness and vertigo plus signs of Yin deficiency.

The tendons and muscles are poorly nourished, because the Liver Yin deficiency fails to control Yang and the deficiency Heat is steaming inside, causing involuntary movement of limbs, dizziness and vertigo, tinnitus, afternoon fever, flushed cheeks, dry mouth and throat, and emaciation. A red tongue without moisture and a thready rapid pulse are the signs of internal deficiency Heat due to Liver Yin deficiency.

Blood deficiency producing Wind

Symptoms: Tremor, twisting of muscles, numbness of limbs, dizziness and vertigo, tinnitus, pallor, pale nails, pale tongue, thready weak pulse.

Pathogenesis: Caused by the malnutrition of tendons and muscles resulting from Blood deficiency due to prolonged disease, and loss of blood in an acute or chronic disease.

Analysis: Symptoms of stirring Wind such as tremor and dizziness and vertigo plus signs of Blood deficiency.

The head, eyes, tendons and muscles, and nails are poorly nourished because of the Liver Blood deficiency, causing tremor, twitching of muscles, numbness of limbs, dizziness and vertigo, tinnitus, pallor, and pale nails. A pale tongue and thready weak pulse are the signs of Blood deficiency.

Differentiation

	Nature	Symptoms
Liver Yang turning into Wind	Upward excess, downward deficiency	Dizziness and vertigo, shaking of the head, tremor, dysphasia, stiff tongue, falling down in a fit with loss of consciousness, hemiplegia. Headache, stiff neck, numbness of the limbs, unsteady walking. Red tongue with a white or sticky coating. Wiry forceful pulse
Extreme Heat producing Wind	Heat	Convulsion, neck rigidity, opisthotonus, upward staring of the eyes, lockjaw. High fever, coma, mania. Deep red tongue. Wiry rapid forceful pulse
Yin deficiency stirring Wind	Deficiency	Involuntary movement of limbs, dizziness and vertigo. Afternoon fever, hot sensation in the Five Centres, dry mouth and throat, emaciation. Red tongue without moisture. Thready rapid pulse
Blood deficiency producing Wind	Deficiency	Tremor, twisting of muscles, spasms and numbness of limbs, dizziness and vertigo. Tinnitus, pallor, pale nails. Pale tongue with white coating. Thready pulse

4.5 Damp Heat in the Liver and Gallbladder, Qi stagnation of the Gallbladder with disturbance of Phlegm

Damp Heat in the Liver and Gallbladder: Manifestations of Liver and Gallbladder disorders in maintaining the free flow of Qi due to accumulation of Damp Heat.

Qi stagnation of the Gallbladder with disturbance of Phlegm: Manifestations of Gallbladder disorders in maintaining the free flow of Qi due to disturbance of Phlegm Heat.

Damp Heat in the Liver and Gallbladder

Symptoms: Hypochondriac distention and pain or masses, poor appetite, abdominal distention, bitter taste in the mouth, nausea, vomiting, abnormal stools, scanty and yellow urine, red tongue, yellow sticky coating, wiry rapid pulse. Or, alternate chills and fever, yellow sclera and skin of the entire body, eczema of the scrotum, swelling and burning pain in the testes, yellow foul leucorrhoea with pruritus vulvae.

Pathogenesis: Invasion of Damp Heat, overeating fatty food causing the production of internal Damp Heat, and disorders of the Spleen in transportation and transformation of food and Water and of the Stomach in receiving food produce Damp, which is transformed into Heat in cases where it stagnates for a long time, thereby causing Damp Heat in the Liver and Gallbladder.

Analysis: Distending pain in the right hypochondrium, poor appetite, yellow urine, red tongue, yellow sticky coating.

Damp Heat causes the Liver to become disordered in keeping the free flow of Qi, causing hypochondriac distention and pain. Qi stagnation with Blood stasis causes the mass. The Liver Wood overacts on the Spleen Earth, causing the failure of Spleen in transportation and transformation, causing anorexia and abdominal distention. The upward going of Stomach-Qi causes the Gallbladder-Qi also to go upward, causing a bitter taste in the mouth. If Damp is greater than Heat, there will be loose stools; when Heat is greater than Damp, there will be dry stools. Damp Heat pours downward, leading to the disordered Qi activity of Bladder, causing scanty and yellow urine. A red tongue with a yellow sticky coating, and wiry rapid pulse are the signs of Damp Heat. The fight between the antipathogenic Qi and pathogenic Qi is the cause of alternate chills and fever. Damp Heat steams the bile and forces it to flow into the skin, causing yellow sclera and skin of the entire body. The downward pouring of Damp Heat affects the perineal region, leading to eczema of the scrotum, swelling and burning pain in the testes, and yellow foul leucorrhoea with pruritus vulvae.

Qi stagnation of the Gallbladder with disturbance of Phlegm

Symptoms: Palpitations due to fright, restlessness, a bitter taste in the mouth, nausea, vomiting, fullness and distention in the hypochondrium, dizziness and vertigo, blurred vision, red tongue with a yellow sticky coating, wiry rolling pulse.

Pathogenesis: With emotional depression, the transformation of Qi stagnation into Fire, which burns and condenses the Body Fluid into Phlegm, is followed by the combination of Phlegm and Heat affecting the Heart and Gallbladder, and as a result, the Gallbladder-Qi and Mind stored in the Heart are disturbed.

Analysis: Palpitation, insomnia, dizziness and vertigo, yellow sticky tongue-coating.

When the Gallbladder is disordered in promoting the free flow of Qi, Qi stagnates, and Phlegm is produced, and the disturbance of Gallbladder-Qi and Mind will be present, causing palpitations and restlessness. Steamed by the Heat, the Gallbladder-Qi goes upward, causing a bitter taste in the mouth. The Gallbladder Heat affects the Stomach, the Qi of which is forced upwards, causing a bitter taste in the mouth, nausea and vomiting. The stagnation of Gallbladder-Qi is manifested as fullness and distention in the hypochondrium. The upward disturbance of Phlegm Heat causes dizziness and vertigo, blurred vision, and tinnitus. A red tongue with a yellow sticky coating, and a wiry rolling pulse are the signs of Phlegm Heat.

5. SYNDROMES OF THE KIDNEYS AND BLADDER

The Kidneys are located at either side of the lumbus. The Kidney Meridian connects with the Bladder, with which it is externally–internally related. The Kidneys store Essence, dominate human reproduction and development, dominate Water metabolism and the reception of Qi, produce marrow to fill up the brain, dominate bone, manufacture Blood, manifest in the hair, open into the ear, and dominate anterior and posterior orifices. The Bladder functions to store and discharge urine.

Diseases of the Kidney

Pathological changes:

1. Abnormality in growth, development and reproduction.

2. Disorders in waste metabolism.

3. Disorders in respiration, insufficiency of brain marrow, and malnutrition of bone, ear and hair.

Symptoms: Soreness and weakness of the lumbus and legs, tinnitus, deafness, loose teeth, falling out of hair, impotence and seminal emission, infertility, sterility, abnormal menstruation, clear and increased volume of urine, enuresis, incontinence of urine, scanty urine, oedema, diarrhoea, asthma with more exhaling and less inhaling.

Deficiency syndromes: Yang deficiency of Kidneys, Yin deficiency of Kidneys, deficiency of Kidney Essence, unconsolidation of Kidney-Qi, failure of Kidneys in receiving Qi.

Diseases of the Bladder

Pathological changes: Disorders of Qi activities of the Bladder with the manifestation of abnormal urination.

Symptoms: Frequent, urgent and painful urination, bloody urine, retention of urine.

Excess syndromes: Damp Heat in the Bladder.

5.1 Deficiency of Kidney Essence, Yin deficiency of Kidneys, Yang deficiency of Kidneys

Deficiency of Kidney Essence: Manifestations of slow development, low ability in reproduction, and senility.

Yin deficiency of the Kidneys: Manifestations of internal Heat.

Yang deficiency of the Kidneys: Manifestations of disturbance in Qi activities due to the failure of Kidney Yang to warm the body.

Deficiency of Kidney Essence

Symptoms: Maldevelopment of the body and intelligence, sexual disorders, infertility, sterility, senility, tinnitus, deafness, forgetfulness, dull response, sluggishness, hair falling out, loose teeth.

Pathogenesis: Caused by congenital deficiency, an acquired deficiency, prolonged disease, or sexual indulgence consuming the Kidney Essence.

Analysis: Maldevelopment of the body and intelligence, low ability in reproduction, senility.

The deficient Kidney Essence is not able to produce enough Qi and Blood to nourish the muscles and bones, causing maldevelopment of the body and intelligence, sexual disorder, infertility, sterility, and senility. The deficiency of Kidney Essence causes a low ability in reproduction and hyposexuality. The outward manifestation of the Kidneys is in the hair, and the teeth are the tip of bone, and therefore hair loss and loose teeth are caused by deficient Kidney Essence. Also the Sea of Marrow is not filled up due to the Essence deficiency, causing tinnitus, deafness, forgetfulness, and dull responses. The tendons and muscles lack the nourishment of the Kidney Essence, causing weakness of the legs and sluggishness.

Yin deficiency of the Kidneys

Symptoms: Soreness and weakness of lumbus and legs, dizziness, tinnitus, insomnia, dream-disturbed sleep, seminal emissions, prospermia, amenorrhoea, uterine functional bleeding, emaciation, afternoon fever, night sweating, a hot sensation in the palms and soles, a dry throat, flushed cheeks, yellow urine, dry stools, red tongue with little coating, a thready rapid pulse.

Pathogenesis: Prolonged consumptive disease consuming the Yin of the Kidneys, exhaustion of Kidney Yin in the late stage of a febrile disease, sexual indulgence damaging the Kidney Yin.

Analysis: Symptoms of Kidney disease plus symptoms of deficiency Heat.

Kidney Yin is deficient, and so the marrow will be reduced and the bones weak, causing soreness and weakness of the lumbus and legs. The brain marrow is reduced, causing symptoms such as dizziness and tinnitus. The harmonious relationship between the Heart and the Kidneys is disturbed, with the Heart Fire flaring, and this leads to insomnia and dream-disturbed sleep. The consolidation of sperm is weakened, and so there is seminal emission and prospermia. Yin deficiency causes the poor production of Blood, leading to amenorrhoea. The deficiency Heat forces Blood to be extravasated, causing uterine functional bleeding. The deficiency Heat from the Kidney Yin deficiency causes emaciation, afternoon fever, night sweating, a hot sensation in the palms and soles, a dry throat, flushed cheeks, yellow urine, dry stools, a red tongue with little coating, and a thready rapid pulse.

Yang deficiency of the Kidneys

Symptoms: Soreness and weakness of the lumbus and legs, cold limbs, pallor or dark complexion, listlessness, dizziness, pale flabby tongue with a white coating, a deep thready weak pulse, impotence, sterility, diarrhoea at dawn with undigested food in the stools, scanty urine, oedema, palpitations, cough, asthma.

Pathogenesis: Constitutional Yang deficiency, Kidney deficiency due to old age, damage of the Kidneys due to prolonged diseases, overindulgence in sexual activities causing the Kidney Yang to become insufficient.

Analysis: Hypofunction of the whole body plus Cold.

The lumbus is known as the house of the Kidneys, which dominates bone. When Kidney Yang is deficient, the lumbus and bones lack warmth and nourishment, causing soreness and weakness of the lumbus and legs and cold limbs. The Heart Shen-Mind is not activated because the Yang Qi is deficient, causing listlessness and dizziness. Qi and Blood are not ample enough to nourish the face, resulting in pallor. When Yang is extremely deficient, turbid Yin is diffuse in skin, causing a dark complexion. A pale flabby tongue with a white coating, and a deep thready weak pulse are signs of weakness of the Qi and Blood circulation due to Kidney Yang deficiency. The Kidneys dominate reproduction, and so hypofunction of reproduction, impotence, and infertility will appear when Kidney Yang is deficient. Failure of Fire to produce Earth causes the dysfunction of Spleen, causing diarrhoea at dawn with undigested food in the stools. The Bladder is disordered in Qi activity due to Kidney Yang deficiency, and so there will be retention of water, causing oedema. Water invades the Heart, causing Heart Yang deficiency, which causes palpitations. The Water affects the Lungs, causing cough and asthma.

5.2 Unconsolidation of Kidney-Qi, failure of the Kidneys in receiving Qi

Unconsolidation of Kidney-Qi: Manifestations of failure of the Kidneys in storing and controlling Essence.

Failure of the Kidneys in receiving Qi: Manifestations of shortness of breath and asthmatic breathing caused by the failure of the Kidneys in receiving Qi.

These two syndromes have the following symptoms in common: soreness and weakness of the lumbus and legs, tinnitus, deafness, listlessness, pale tongue with a white coating, weak pulse.

Unconsolidation of Kidney-Qi

Symptoms: Pallor, listlessness, decline in hearing, soreness and weakness of the lumbus and legs, frequent urination with clear and increased volume of urine, dribbling of urine, enuresis, incontinence of urine, spermatorrhoea, premature ejaculation, prolonged menstrual flow, Cold leucorrhoea in big quantities, pale tongue with a white coating, deep weak pulse.

Pathogenesis: Kidney-Qi deficiency in old age, congenital deficiency, prolonged disease damaging the Kidney-Qi.

Analysis: Symptoms of the Kidneys and Bladder failing to store.

The Kidneys are deficient and so the ear is not well nourished, causing a decline in hearing. The bones lack nourishment from the Kidney-Qi, causing soreness and weakness of lumbus and legs. The Bladder is out of control because the Kidneys are deficient, causing frequent urination with a clear and increased volume of urine, the dribbling of urine, enuresis, and incontinence of urine. The Kidneys store Essence and so when the Kidney-Qi is deficient, the control of sperm is damaged, causing spermatorrhoea and premature ejaculation, prolonged menstrual flow, and Cold leucorrhoea in large quantities. A pale tongue, with a white coating, and a deep weak pulse are the signs of Kidney-Qi deficiency.

Failure of the Kidneys in receiving Qi

Symptoms: Asthmatic breathing, shortness of breath manifested as more exhaling and less inhaling and aggravated on exertion, spontaneous sweating, tiredness, a low voice, soreness and weakness of the lumbus and legs, a pale tongue with a white coating, a deep weak pulse. Or dyspnoea, profuse Cold sweating, cold limbs, a blue complexion, and a floating pulse without root. Or abrupt breathing, a red face, irritability, dry throat, red tongue and a thready rapid pulse.

Pathogenesis: Prolonged cough and asthma consume the Lung-Qi and later involve the Kidneys. Or overwork causes deficiency of Qi, leading to the loss of function of the Kidneys in receiving Qi.

Analysis: Prolonged cough and asthma, more exhaling and less inhaling, worse on exertion plus symptoms of Qi deficiency of the Lungs and Kidneys.

The Kidneys fail to receive Qi, causing asthmatic breathing, and shortness of breath manifested as more exhaling and less inhaling and aggravated on exertion. The bones are deprived of nourishment, causing soreness and weakness of the lumbus and legs. The Lung-Qi is deficient and so the body defence will be weak, causing spontaneous sweating. Hypofunction causes tiredness and a faint voice. A pale tongue with a white coating, and a deep weak pulse are the signs of Qi deficiency. If Yang Qi is collapsed, there will be dyspnoea, profuse Cold sweating, cold limbs, and a blue complexion. If the deficiency of Yang goes outward, a floating pulse without root will appear. A prolonged Qi deficiency of the Kidneys makes the Kidney Yin deficient as well, consequently the deficiency Fire flares, causing abrupt breathing, a red face, irritability, and a dry throat. A red tongue and thready rapid pulse are the signs of Yin deficiency with internal Heat.

Differentiation

	Nature	Symptoms
Yang deficiency of the Kidneys	Deficiency	Soreness and weakness of the lumbus and legs, cold limbs, impotence, infertility, sterility, diarrhoea at dawn, oedema. A pale flabby tongue with a white coating. Deep weak pulse
Yin deficiency of the Kidneys	Deficiency	Soreness and weakness of the lumbus and legs, insomnia, dream-disturbed sleep, seminal emission, prospermia, afternoon fever, night sweating, dry throat, flushed cheeks, yellow urine, dry stools. Red tongue with little coating. Thready rapid pulse
Deficiency of Kidney Essence	Deficiency	Flaccidity, oligospermia, amenorrhoea, hair falling out, loose teeth, poor memory, deafness, sluggishness, flaccid lower limbs, slow responses. Reddish tongue, white coating. Deep thready pulse
Unconsolidation of Kidney-Qi	Deficiency	Soreness and weakness of lumbus and legs, decline in hearing, frequent urination with clear and increased volume of urine, dribbling of urine, enuresis, incontinence of urine, spermatorrhoea, premature ejaculation. Pale tongue with white coating. Deep weak pulse
Failure of the Kidneys in receiving Qi	Deficiency	Asthmatic breathing, shortness of breath manifested as more exhaling and less inhaling and aggravated on exertion, spontaneous sweating, tiredness, low voice, soreness and weakness of lumbus and legs. Pale tongue with a white coating. Deep weak pulse

5.3 Damp Heat in the Bladder

This refers to those manifestations of the disturbed Qi activity of the Bladder in abnormal urination.

Symptoms: Frequent, urgent and painful urination, dark yellow and scanty urine, distending pain in the lower abdomen. Or fever, lumbar pain, bloody urine, sandy urine. Red tongue with a yellow sticky coating, rapid pulse.

Pathogenesis: The disordered Qi activity of the Bladder results from invasion of Damp Heat, or improper food producing internal Damp Heat, which pours down to the Bladder.

Analysis: Frequent, urgent and painful urination, yellow urine.

Frequent, urgent and painful urination is from the invasion of Damp Heat to the Bladder. Dark yellow and scanty urine and a distending pain in the lower abdomen are the result of disorders of the Qi activity of the Bladder. bloody urine occurs because of the damage to the vessels of the Bladder. Sandy urine is due to the concentration of the substance of urine by Heat. A red tongue with a yellow sticky coating and a rapid pulse are the signs of Damp Heat.

6. COMPLICATED SYNDROMES OF THE ZANG FU ORGANS

The complicated syndromes of the Zang Fu organs are those in which two organs or more are diseased at the same time, or in succession.

6.1 Qi deficiency of Heart and Lungs, deficiency of Heart and Spleen, Blood deficiency of Heart and Liver

Qi deficiency of Heart and Lungs: Manifestations of Qi deficiency of both Heart and Lungs.

Deficiency of Heart and Spleen: Manifestations of Blood deficiency of Heart and Qi deficiency of Spleen.

Blood deficiency of Heart and Liver: Manifestations of Blood deficiency of both Heart and Liver.

These three syndromes have the following symptoms in common: palpitation, listlessness, pallor, dizziness, pale tongue, white coating.

Qi deficiency of Heart and Lungs

Symptoms: Palpitations, cough in a low voice that becomes worse on exertion, shortness of breath, fullness in the chest, clear and thin Phlegm, pale complexion, dizziness, listlessness, spontaneous sweating, low voice. Pale tongue with white coating, deep weak or knotted pulse.

Pathogenesis: Prolonged cough exhausts Qi of the Heart and Lungs. Congenital deficiency or weak constitution due to old age can cause Qi deficiency of the Lungs, the production of pectoral Qi will be deficient and so there will be Qi deficiency of the Heart. Where Qi of the Heart is deficient, the pectoral Qi will vanish, causing Qi deficiency of the Lungs.

Analysis: Palpitation, cough, plus symptoms of Qi deficiency.

Heart-Qi deficiency produces palpitations. Lung-Qi deficiency leading to the failure of Lung-Qi in descending produces a cough. Qi deficiency produces shortness of breath, which becomes worse on exertion. Lung-Qi deficiency leading to weakened respiration produces fullness in the chest. Retention of Body Fluid produces clear and thin Phlegm. Hypofunction of the whole body due to Qi deficiency produces a pale complexion, dizziness, and listlessness. Unconsolidation of Wei-defence produces spontaneous sweating. Insufficiency of pectoral Qi produces low voice. A pale tongue with a white coating and a deep weak or knotted pulse are the signs of Qi and Blood deficiency.

Deficiency of Heart and Spleen

Symptoms: Palpitation, insomnia, dream-disturbed sleep, dizziness, forgetfulness, sallow complexion, listlessness, subcutaneous bleeding, decreased menstrual flow, which is pale in colour and longer in duration. Pale tender tongue, and thready weak pulse.

Pathogenesis: Prolonged disease, overwork or chronic haemorrhage can cause deficiency of both the Heart and the Spleen. With the Spleen-Qi deficiency, poor production of Blood and failure of the Spleen in controlling Blood, there will be extravasation of Blood, causing Heart Blood deficiency. With Heart Blood deficiency, Qi production will be without substance and thus the Spleen-Qi will also be deficient.

Analysis: Palpitations, insomnia, sallow complexion, poor appetite, abdominal distention, loose stools, chronic haemorrhage plus symptoms of Qi and Blood deficiency.

Heart Blood deficiency produces palpitations. The Mind is disturbed, causing insomnia and dream-disturbed sleep. The head and eyes are deprived of nourishment, leading to dizziness and forgetfulness. The skin without nourishment looks lustreless, resulting in a sallow complexion. The transportation and transformation of the Spleen is not normal owing to the Spleen-Qi deficiency, showing as abdominal distention and loose stools. Hypofunction due to Qi deficiency produces listlessness. The subcutaneous bleeding and scanty menstruation indicate the dysfunction of the Spleen in controlling Blood. A pale tender tongue and thready weak pulse are the signs of Qi and Blood deficiency.

Blood deficiency of Heart and Liver

Symptoms: Palpitations, insomnia, dream-disturbed sleep, dizziness, tinnitus, pallor, blurred vision with a dry sensation in the eyes, pale nails, numbness of the limbs, tremor, spasms of the tendons, scanty menstrual flow or amenorrhoea. Pale tongue with a white coating, and a weak pulse.

Pathogenesis: Weak constitution due to prolonged disease, or worries and over-thinking consuming Yin Blood can cause Heart Blood deficiency, in which the Liver has not enough Blood to store and therefore the Liver does not function in regulating the volume of Blood in vessels.

Analysis: Palpitations, insomnia, eyes and tendons lack nourishment, plus symptoms of Blood deficiency.

Heart Blood deficiency produces palpitations. The Mind is disturbed, causing insomnia and dream-disturbed sleep. The head is deprived of the nourishment of Blood, leading to dizziness, tinnitus, and pallor. The eyes do not get enough nourishment from the Liver Blood, so there is blurred vision with a dry sensation in the eyes. The muscles and tendons don't have enough nourishment from the Liver Blood, producing pale nails, numbness of the limbs, tremor, and spasms of the tendons. Scanty menstrual flow and amenorrhoea come from the Liver Blood deficiency. A pale tongue with a white coating and weak pulse are the signs of Blood deficiency.

6.2 Yang deficiency of Heart and Kidneys, Yang deficiency of Spleen and Kidneys

Yang deficiency of Heart and Kidneys: Manifestations of Yang deficiency of both Heart and Kidneys with interior Cold.

Yang deficiency of Spleen and Kidneys: Manifestations of Yang deficiency of both Spleen and Kidneys.

These two syndomes have the following symptoms in common: pallor, cold limbs, oedema, scanty urine. Pale tender tongue with a white slippery coating, deep thready pulse.

Yang deficiency of Heart and Kidneys

Symptoms: Palpitations, cold limbs, sleepiness, scanty urine, oedema (especially of lower limbs), bluish lips and nails, pale dark or purplish tongue with a white slippery coating, deep weak thready pulse.

Pathogenesis: Prolonged disease causes damage to the Yang of the Heart and Kidneys, producing the internal Cold and hypofunction of the whole body, and consequently Blood stasis and retention of water are present.

Analysis: Palpitations, oedema, scanty urine plus symptoms of deficiency Cold.

With the Heart Yang deficiency, the Mind lacks nourishment, causing palpitations and sleepiness. Without the warmth given by the Heart Yang, there will be cold limbs. The Qi activity of the Bladder is low in function and the symptoms of this are scanty urine and oedema, especially of the lower limbs. Yang deficiency causes Blood stagnation, resulting in bluish lips and nails. A pale dark or purplish tongue with a white slippery coating and a deep weak thready pulse are the signs of Blood stasis from the Yang deficiency of Heart and Kidneys.

Yang deficiency of Spleen and Kidneys

Symptoms: Pallor, cold limbs, Cold pain in the lumbus, knees and lower abdomen, prolonged diarrhoea, diarrhoea at dawn with undigested food in stools, scanty urine, oedema, abdominal distention. Pale tender tongue with white slippery coating, deep thready pulse.

Pathogenesis: Either prolonged disease damaging the Yang Qi of the Spleen and Kidneys, or prolonged diarrhoea in which the diseased Spleen involves the Kidneys, or a Yang deficiency of the Kidneys causes Water flushing in which the diseased Kidneys involve the Spleen, producing Yang deficiency of both, so that the warming and Qi activity of the Kidneys do not work.

Analysis: Cold pain, prolonged diarrhoea, oedema plus symptoms of deficiency Cold.

Yang deficiency gives no warmth to the body, causing pallor, cold limbs, and a cold pain in the lumbus and knees. The internal Cold also causes a cold pain in the lower abdomen. The Fire of the Mingmen is weakened by Yang deficiency, causing prolonged diarrhoea and diarrhoea at dawn. Water and food are not warmed by Yang because it is deficient and this causes diarrhoea with undigested food in the stools. In the case of Yang deficiency, Qi activity of the Bladder is not active in warming and discharging Water, which then flows to the skin causing oedema. Earth fails to act on Water and, on the contrary, is acted upon by Water, causing abdominal distention. A pale tender tongue with a white slippery coating and a deep thready pulse are the signs of Yang deficiency with excessive Water Cold in the interior.

6.3 Disharmony between Heart and Kidneys, Yin deficiency of Liver and Kidneys, Yin deficiency of Lungs and Kidneys

Disharmony between Heart and Kidneys: Manifestations of the breakdown of the harmonious relationship between the Heart and the Kidneys.

Yin deficiency of Liver and Kidneys: Manifestations of Yin deficiency of both Liver and Kidneys.

Yin deficiency of Lungs and Kidneys: Manifestations of Yin fluid deficiency of both Lungs and Kidneys.

These three syndromes have the following symptoms in common: soreness and weakness of lumbus and knees, seminal emission, dry throat, hot sensation in palms and soles, tidal fever, night sweating, a red tongue with little or no coating, and a thready rapid pulse.

Disharmony between Heart and Kidneys

Symptoms: Irritability, insomnia, palpitations, dizziness, tinnitus, forgetfulness, soreness and weakness of lumbus and legs, seminal emission, hot sensation in the Five Centres, dry throat. Red tongue with a little coating, thready rapid pulse.

Pathogenesis: Prolonged disease, sexual indulgence, anxiety and over-thinking; Fire transformed from emotional depression, invasion of exogenous Fire, and excessive Heart Fire can cause Yin deficiency of Heart and Kidneys, leading to hyperactivity of Yang, through which the harmonious relationship between the Heart and the Kidneys is broken down.

Analysis: Insomnia plus symptoms of Heart Fire hyperactivity and Kidney Water deficiency.

The Heart Yang is in a state of hyperactivity because of the failure of the harmonious relationship between the Heart and the Kidneys, and the symptoms that follow the Mind being disturbed will include irritability, insomnia, and palpitations. In cases where the brain is without adequate nourishment as a result of Yin deficiency of the Kidneys, there will be dizziness, tinnitus, and forgetfulness. The lumbus lacking nourishment due to the Kidney Yin deficiency is disturbed, with the deficiency Fire affecting the store of Essence and causing the soreness and weakness of the lumbus and legs, seminal emission, hot sensation in the Five

Centres, and a dry throat. A red tongue and a thready rapid pulse are signs of Water deficiency and Fire hyperactivity.

Yin deficiency of Liver and Kidneys

Symptoms: Dizziness, blurred vision, tinnitus, poor memory, insomnia, dream-disturbed sleep, dry throat, soreness and weakness of the lumbus and legs, hypochondriac pain, hot sensation in the palms and soles, flushed cheeks, night sweating, seminal emission, scanty menstrual flow, red tongue with little coating and a thready rapid pulse.

Pathogenesis: Prolonged disease, sexual indulgence, and emotional damage exhausting the Yin Essence, leading to Yin deficiency causing the disturbance by deficiency Fire.

Analysis: Tinnitus, seminal emission, insomnia, soreness and weakness of the lumbus and legs, hypochondriac pain plus symptoms of Yin deficiency with internal Heat.

Dizziness, blurred vision, tinnitus, and poor memory are due to Yin deficiency and Yang hyperactivity. Insomnia and dream-disturbed sleep are the result of the disturbance of Mind stored in the Heart by the internal deficiency Heat. Dry throat and soreness and weakness of the lumbus and legs develop from Kidney Yin deficiency. Hypochondriac pain comes from the malnutrition of the Liver Meridian due to Liver Yin deficiency. The hot sensation in the palms and soles, and flushed cheeks result from the Yin deficiency causing internal Heat. The Heat forces the Body Fluid to go outward, causing night sweating. Seminal emission comes from disturbance of the store of Essence. Chong and Ren are empty due to Yin deficiency of Liver and Kidneys, producing scanty menstrual flow. A red tongue with little coating and a thready rapid pulse are the signs of Yin deficiency producing internal Heat.

Yin deficiency of Lungs and Kidneys

Symptoms: Unproductive cough or cough with a small amount of sputum or Blood-tinged sputum, dry throat, hoarseness, emaciation, soreness and weakness of the lumbus and legs, steaming Heat in bones, tidal fever, flushed cheeks, night sweating, seminal emission, irregular menstruation. Red tongue with little coating, thready rapid pulse.

Pathogenesis: Prolonged cough causes Yin deficiency of Lungs and later involves the Kidneys. Kidney Yin deficiency, or Kidney Yin gets exhausted by sexual indulgence and later involves the Lungs.

Analysis: Prolonged cough with Blood-tinged sputum, soreness and weakness of lumbus and knees, seminal emission plus symptoms of Yin deficiency.

Unproductive cough or cough with a small amount of sputum or Blood-tinged sputum comes from the deficiency Fire burning the Lung vessels due to Lung Yin deficiency. Dry throat and hoarseness result from the deficiency Fire burning the Body Fluid. Emaciation indicates poor nourishment of muscles and soreness and weakness of the lumbus and knees is because of poor nourishment from the Yin deficiency of the Kidneys. A feeling of steaming Heat in the bones and tidal fever are due to internal Heat. Night sweating comes from disturbance of Ying-nutrient by the flaring of deficiency Fire. Seminal emission implies the disturbance of the store of Essence from Heat. Scanty menstrual flow is because of the Blood deficiency.

6.4 Imbalance between the Liver and Spleen, Disharmony between the Liver and Stomach

Imbalance between the Liver and Spleen: Manifestations of disorders of the Liver in keeping free flow of Qi, and of Spleen in transportation and transformation.

Disharmony between the Liver and Stomach: Manifestations of disorders of the Liver in keeping free flow of Qi, and of Stomach-Qi in descending.

These two syndromes have the following symptoms in common: distending pain in the hypochondrium and epigastrium, mental depression or irritability, wiry pulse.

Imbalance between the Liver and Spleen

Symptoms: Distending pain in the hypochondrium and chest, sighing, mental depression or irritability, poor appetite, abdominal distention, loose stools, borborygmus, flatulence, abdominal pain. White sticky tongue-coating, wiry pulse.

Pathogenesis: Emotional depression and anger damage the Liver, known as 'Wood stagnation over-acting on Earth', which loses its function in transportation and transformation. Improper diet and overwork injure the Spleen, and when its normal function is lost, it then counteracts on the Liver Wood.

Analysis: Poor appetite, abdominal distention, loose stools, distending pain in the hypochondrium and chest.

It is Qi stagnation coming from the dysfunction of the Liver in keeping a free flow of Qi that causes the distending pain in the hypochondrium and chest. Sighing occurs because it can relieve Qi stagnation. Qi stagnation causes mental depression or irritability, and Qi stagnation and Damp retention bring on poor appetite, abdominal distention, loose stools, borborygmus and flatulence. Qi stagnation gets better on discharge of stools, causing relief of abdominal pain. A white sticky tongue-coating is the sign of Damp on the inside and the wiry pulse refers to the Liver disorders.

Disharmony between the Liver and Stomach

Symptoms: Distending pain in the hypochondrium and epigastrium, belching, hiccups, acid regurgitation, irritability, a red tongue with thin yellow coating, wiry rapid pulse. Or headache, which is made worse by exposure to cold and better by warmth, watery vomiting, and cold limbs. Pale tongue, white slippery coating, deep wiry tense pulse.

Pathogenesis:

1. Emotional depression and Qi stagnation transforming into Fire affect the Stomach, presenting symptoms including distending pain in the epigastrium and hypochondrium and acid regurgitation.

2. Invasion of Cold to the Liver and Stomach presents symptoms including headaches at the top of the head, watery vomiting, and a white slippery tongue-coating.

Analysis: The Liver Fire affects the Stomach and then causes Qi stagnation of the Liver and Stomach, causing distending pain in the hypochondrium and epigastrium. The Stomach-Qi goes upward abnormally, causing belching and hiccuping. Qi and Fire of Liver and Stomach obstruct in the inside, causing acid regurgitation. The Liver loses its normal function in keeping a free flow of Qi, causing irritability. A red tongue with a thin yellow coating, and a wiry rapid pulse are signs of Qi stagnation transforming into Fire.

Pathogenic Cold invades the Liver and Stomach and goes along the Liver Meridian to the top of head and gets blocked there, causing a headache at the top of the head. Cold is a Yin pathogenic factor and is characterized by contraction, which aggravates the headache. The damage of the Yang of the Middle Burner causes the water retention and upward movement of Qi, leading to watery vomiting. Cold injures Yang Qi, causing cold limbs. A pale tongue with a white slippery coating and a deep wiry tense pulse are signs of Cold retention in the inside.

6.5 Qi deficiency of the Spleen and Lungs, invasion of the Lungs by Liver Fire

Qi deficiency of the Spleen and Lungs: Manifestations of the Qi deficiency of both Spleen and Lungs.

Invasion of the Lungs by the Liver Fire: Manifestations of the Qi and Fire of the Liver Meridian affecting the Lungs.

Qi deficiency of the Spleen and Lungs

Symptoms: Prolonged cough, shortness of breath, profuse thin white sputum, poor appetite, abdominal distention, loose stools, low voice, tiredness, oedema of face and feet. Pale tongue with a white coating and a thready weak pulse.

Pathogenesis: Prolonged cough causes Qi deficiency of the Lungs and then involves the Spleen. Improper diet and overwork damage the function of the Spleen and then involve the Lungs. The Spleen-Qi deficiency produces its failure in transportation and transformation, and the Lungs then fail to dominate Qi for respiration and for the whole body.

Analysis: Poor appetite, abdominal distention, loose stools, prolonged cough, plus symptoms of Qi deficiency.

Lung-Qi is damaged by the prolonged cough. Qi deficiency causes the Body Fluid to be maldistributed, and Phlegm is produced by accumulation of Damp, causing profuse thin white sputum. The Spleen is disordered in transportation and transformation due to its Qi deficiency, causing poor appetite, abdominal distention, and loose stools. Qi deficiency causes the decline of functional activities, resulting in low voice and tiredness. The Water Damp is strong, causing oedema of face and feet. A pale tongue with a white coating, and a thready weak pulse are the signs of Qi deficiency.

Invasion of the Lungs by Liver Fire

Symptoms: Burning pain in the hypochondrium, irritability, dizziness, redness of the eyes, bitter taste in the mouth, cough with a small amount of yellow sticky sputum or even haemoptysis. Red tongue with a thin yellow coating, and a wiry rapid pulse.

Pathogenesis: Anger damages the Liver, Qi stagnation of which transforms into Fire. The Liver Fire affects the Lungs, causing them to function abnormally in descending.

Analysis: Cough, burning pain in the hypochondrium, irritability, bitter taste in the mouth plus symptoms of interior excess Heat

The Fire of the Liver Meridian gives rise to a burning pain in the hypochondrium. The Liver loses its function in keeping free flow of Qi, causing irritability. The Liver Fire flares, causing dizziness and redness of the eyes. Stagnation of Qi and Fire steams the bile, causing a bitter taste in the mouth. The Qi and Fire go upward to affect the Lung Metal, burning the fluid into Phlegm, leading to a cough with a small amount of yellow sticky sputum. The Lung vessels are damaged by the Fire, which causes haemoptysis. A red tongue with a thin yellow coating, and wiry rapid pulse are the signs of the excess Fire of the Liver Meridian.

V. DIFFERENTIATION OF SYNDROMES ACCORDING TO THE THEORY OF THE SIX MERIDIANS

This is a differentiation method in which the manifestation of a febrile disease is classified into Taiyang disease, Yangming disease, and Shaoyang disease, known as the Three Yang diseases, and Taiyin disease, Shaoyin disease, and Jueyin disease, known as the Three Yin diseases. The characteristics of pathological changes are analyzed according to the nature of the struggle between the antipathogenic Qi and pathogenic Qi, the location of disease, and the development tendency of the various stages in the disease. Created by Dr Zhang Zhongjing of the Eastern Han dynasty, this method lays the foundation for the differentiation of syndromes in TCM.

1. TAIYANG SYNDROME

Taiyang meridians are the most superficial, playing a role in protecting the body like a fence. When the pathogenic factors invade, mostly entering the body from Taiyang Meridians, the antipathogenic Qi rises spiritedly to struggle with the pathogenic factors – in the process of which, Taiyang disease occurs.

Taiyang Jing-Meridian syndrome

This is due to the invasion of pathogenic Wind Cold to the Taiyang Meridian, causing the disorders of Ying-nutrient and Wei-defence, usually seen in the initial stage of the infection and marked by chills and fever, pain of the neck, and a superficial pulse. This includes Attack of Taiyang Meridian by Wind and by Cold.

A. Attack of Taiyang Meridian by Wind

Manifested by strong Wei but weak Ying, the Attack of Taiyang Meridian by Wind is symptomized as fever, aversion to Wind, sweating, superficial and a rather slow pulse, nose noises and retching.

B. Attack of Taiyang Meridian by Cold

Manifested by inhibited Wei-Yang and stagnated Ying-Yin, the Attack of Taiyang Meridian by Cold is symptomized as fever, aversion to cold, pain of the neck, aching all over the body, a lack of sweating, and a superficial and tense pulse.

Taiyang Fu-organ syndrome

This is the pathogenic condition in which the pathogen of Taiyang Meridian syndrome is transmitted to the Bladder (Taiyang Fu-organ), including the syndromes of Taiyang Water-storing and Blood-storing.

A. Syndrome of Taiyang Water-storing

This is the pathogenic condition in which the pathogen of Taiyang Meridian syndrome is blocked in the Bladder, causing retention of water, manifested as fever, aversion to cold, scanty urine, fullness in the lower abdomen, thirst, vomiting of water after drinking, and superficial pulse or superficial and rapid pulse.

B. Syndrome of Taiyang Blood-storing

This is the pathogenic condition in which the pathogen of Taiyang Meridian syndrome is transmitted to the lower abdomen and stagnates with Blood, being manifest as hardness and fullness of the lower abdomen, mental mania, forgetfulness, black stools, and a deep and hesitant pulse.

2. YANGMING SYNDROME

In the progress of exogenous febrile disease, the excessive Heat causes dryness and Heat in the Stomach and intestines. This is the syndrome caused by the transmission of the pathogen of Taiyang Meridian syndrome to the Yangming Meridian and changed to Heat; or is caused by the transmission of the Heat of Shaoyang disease to Yangming; or caused by the transmission of the pathogenic factor to the interior and changing into Heat on the base of an excessive Heat constitution.

Clinical symptoms are fever, aversion to heat, sweating, and a big pulse.

Yangming Jing-Meridian syndrome

This is a pathogenic condition in which the extreme Heat in the Yangming Meridian diffuses to the whole body, but without dry faeces in the intestines.

Clinical symptoms: High fever, profuse sweating, extreme thirst with a desire to drink, irritability, restlessness, coarse breathing, red face, yellow and dry tongue-coating, surging pulse.

Yangming Fu-organ syndrome

This is a pathogenic condition in which the extreme Heat in Yangming Meridian stagnates with the wastes in the intestines, causing the formation of dry faeces in the intestines.

Clinical symptoms: Afternoon fever, sweating of hands and feet, abdominal pain and fullness that is worse on pressure, constipation, coma with delirium, restlessness, sleeplessness, a yellow thick dry and thorny or even burnt black tongue-coating, deep and forceful or rolling and rapid pulse.

3. SHAOYANG SYNDROME

This is the syndrome that shows the pathological changes of the exogenous relationship between the exterior and the interior, in which the Gallbladder is affected by pathogenic factors, resulting in stagnation of Qi. It is mostly developed from the Taiyang Meridian syndrome, and the pathogenic factor is transmitted to Shaoyang, the half exterior and the half interior part of the body, or from the Jueyin syndrome coming to Shaoyang.

Clinical symptoms: Bitter taste in mouth, dry throat, blurred vision, alternate fever and chills, fullness of the chest and hypochondrium, loss of appetite, dysphoria, nausea and/or vomiting, and a taut pulse.

4. TAIYIN SYNDROME

This is a Spleen Yang Deficiency syndrome with the manifestations of Cold Damp caused by damage of the Spleen Yang during improper treatment for Three Yang diseases, or direct invasion of Wind Cold.

Clinical symptoms: Abdominal pain and distention, vomiting, diarrhoea, deep retarded and weak pulse.

5. SHAOYIN SYNDROME

This is a syndrome in which the Yin and Yang of the whole body has declined, and is characterized by deficiency symptoms of the Heart and Kidneys, such as thready pulse and sleepiness.

Cold-type changes of Shaoyin

This refers to the pathological changes of Cold type due to a deficiency of Yang of the Heart and Kidneys during the advanced stage of a febrile disease.

Clinical symptoms: Aversion to cold, sleepiness, cold limbs, thready weak pulse, diarrhoea, vomiting, or fever without aversion to cold, and possibly red face.

Heat-type changes of Shaoyin

This refers to the pathological changes of Heat type due to deficiency of Yin of the Heart and Kidneys with relatively excessive Heart Fire at the advanced stage of a febrile disease.

Clinical symptoms: Dysphoria, insomnia, dry and sore throat, deep red tongue and thready rapid pulse.

6. JUEYIN SYNDROME

This refers to the final stage of febrile disease, with the complicated manifestations of Cold and Heat (mainly upper-Heat and lower-Cold), in which Yin and Yang are at their turning point of transformation.

Clinical symptoms: Thirst, epigastric distress and burning sensation, hunger but no desire for eating, even vomiting of ascaris.

7. TRANSMISSION BETWEEN MERIDIANS

He-combination: Simultaneous involvement of two or three meridians.

Bing-complication: Febrile disease with symptoms of two meridians appearing in sequence with partial overlap.

Chuan-transmission:

- The ordered transmission is in the sequence from Taiyang to Yangming to Shaoyang to Taiyin to Shaoyin to Jueyin.
- The skip-over transmission is skipping over one or more of the meridians, not in the sequence of the six meridians.
- The exterior–interior transmission is the progress of febrile disease from–to the exterior–interior meridians.

Zhi Zhong-direct attack: In the regular pattern of transmission of acute febrile disease, the three Yang meridians are affected first, followed by the three Yin meridians. But when the pathogenic factors are prevailing and the antipathogenic Qi is weak, the pathogenic Cold may attack the three Yin meridians directly.

VI. DIFFERENTIATION OF SYNDROMES ACCORDING TO THE THEORY OF WEI-DEFENCE, QI, YING-NUTRIENT AND XUE-BLOOD

Established by Ye Tianshi of the Qing dynasty, this is a method to differentiate the development of an epidemic febrile disease by studying conditions of the four systems: Wei-defence, Qi, Ying-nutrient and Xue-Blood.

1. WEIFEN SYNDROME

The pathogenic factor of epidemic febrile disease affects the Lungs, causing disorders of the Lungs in dispersing. This is the initial stage of epidemic febrile disease, manifested by fever, slight aversion to Wind and Cold, redness of the tip and edge of the tongue, and superficial and rapid pulse.

Clinical symptoms: Fever, slight aversion to Wind and Cold, redness of the tip and edge of the tongue, superficial and rapid pulse, accompanied with headache, cough, slight thirst, and sore throat.

2. QIFEN SYNDROME

This is an interior Excess Heat syndrome showing the invasion of excessive Heat with fever, no aversion to Cold, red tongue with yellow coating, and rapid and forceful pulse as its main manifestations.

Clinical symptoms: Fever, aversion to Heat, thirst, sweating, irritability, dark yellow urine, rapid and forceful pulse, accompanied with cough, dyspnoea, chest pain, thick yellow sputum, irritability, restlessness, afternoon fever, abdominal distention and pain that is worse on pressure, delirium, constipation or diarrhoea, yellow dry or even black thorny tongue-coating, deep and forceful pulse, bitter taste in mouth, hypochondriac pain, retching, and a taut and rapid pulse.

3. YINGFEN SYNDROME

This is a serious stage of epidemic febrile disease with the disturbance of the Mind by pathogenic Heat due to development of Qifen syndrome or direct transmission of Weifen syndrome to the Pericardium, or a serious febrile disease occurring in the case of deficiency of Ying-Yin in constitution.

Clinical symptoms: Fever higher at night, no thirst, irritability or delirium, sleeplessness, faint skin rashes, dark red tongue without coating, and thready and rapid pulse.

4. XUEFEN SYNDROME

This is a critical stage of epidemic febrile disease usually transmitted from the Yingfen syndrome, manifested by exhaustion of Yin, stirring up of the Wind, and bleeding. The organs mainly involved are the Heart, Liver and Kidneys in this stage.

Clinical symptoms:

1. *Xuefen Excess Heat*: Fever higher at night, restlessness or even manic mental disorders, haematemesis, epistaxis, haematochezia, skin rashes in a dark purple colour, a dark red tongue, a thready and rapid pulse, or convulsions, opisthotonus, up-staring of eyes, trismus, cold limbs, and a taut and rapid pulse.

2. *Xuefen Deficiency Heat*: Low fever, higher at night and lower in morning, hot sensation in palms and soles, listlessness, sleepiness, deafness, emaciation, thready and weak pulse, or involuntary movement of the limbs.

5. TRANSMISSION BETWEEN SYNDROMES

Sequential transmission: An epidemic febrile disease transmitting from Weifen, to Qifen, Yingfen, and Xuefen, indicating the progress from mild to serious, from excess to deficiency.

Reverse transmission: Transmission from Weifen to Yingfen or Xuefen, indicating a critical condition.

Syndrome of both Weifen and Qifen: Pathogenic Heat attacks Qifen while the Weifen syndrome still exists.

Intense Heat in both Qifen and Yingfen or Xuefen: Yingfen or Xuefen syndrome occurs when Qifen syndrome still exists. At the beginning of an epidemic febrile disease, Qifen or Yingfen syndrome occurs directly without manifestation of Weifen syndrome.

VII. DIFFERENTIATION OF SYNDROMES ACCORDING TO THE THEORY OF THE TRIPLE BURNER

This is a differentiation method established by Wu Jutong of the Qing dynasty to differentiate syndromes for treating epidemic febrile diseases, by which the course of disease is divided into Upper Burner, Middle Burner and Lower Burner stages to explain their pathological changes and laws of transmission.

1. SYNDROME OF THE UPPER BURNER

This is the syndrome due to the invasion of the Lung by pathogens at the early stage of an acute febrile disease. In the sequential transmission, the pathogen will be transmitted to the Middle Burner, showing symptoms of the Stomach. In the reverse transmission, the pathogen will be transmitted to the Pericardium, showing symptoms of the Pericardium.

Clinical symptoms: Fever higher in the afternoon, slight aversion to Wind Cold, sweating, thirst or no thirst, cough, superficial and rapid pulse or Cun pulse of both sides being big. In case the pathogen is transmitted to the Pericardium, there will be stiffness of tongue with slurred speech, cold limbs, coma and delirium.

2. SYNDROME OF THE MIDDLE BURNER

This is the middle stage of an epidemic febrile disease, in which the invasion of the Spleen and Stomach by pathogens shows either Yangming Heat damaging Yin or Taiyin Damp Heat.

Clinical symptoms: Fever, red face, coarse breathing, abdominal fullness, constipation, coma and delirium, thirst with a desire for Cold drinks, dry mouth and lips, scanty yellow urine, dry yellow or burnt black tongue-coating, deep and forceful pulse, or recessive fever in which when the patient's skin is felt, it does not feel hot initially but only does so after being felt for a rather long time, heaviness and pain of the body and head, fullness in the epigastric region, nausea, loose stools, a yellow and sticky tongue-coating, and a thready soft and rapid pulse.

3. SYNDROME OF THE LOWER BURNER

This refers to the later stage of an epidemic febrile disease when the Liver and Kidneys are impaired.

Clinical symptoms: Fever, flushed cheeks, listlessness, deafness, a hot sensation in the palms and soles worse than in the dorsum of the hands and feet, dry throat, big and weak pulse, involuntary movement of limbs, palpitations, listlessness, dark red tongue with little coating, or even collapse.

4. TRANSMISSION BETWEEN THE BURNERS

Sequential transmission: From Upper Burner to Middle Burner and Lower Burner, indicating the progress of the febrile disease from superficial to deep, and from mild to serious.

Reverse transmission: From the Lungs to the Pericardium, indicating that the pathogenic Heat is excessive and the disease is serious.

In addition, one can sometimes observe conditions where the Upper Burner syndrome is cured without transmission to Middle Burner; the Middle Burner syndrome occurs when the Upper Burner syndrome still exists; the transmission from Upper Burner is directly to Lower Burner; the Lower Burner syndrome occurs when the Middle Burner syndrome still exists; the Lower Burner syndrome appears from the beginning of the diseases the syndromes of two Burners react with each other; or even three Burners are involved simultaneously.

HOW TO WRITE CASE REPORTS

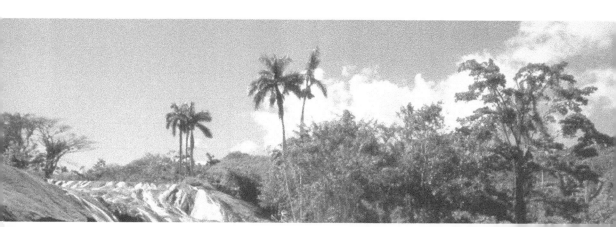

A TCM Case Report is the record of general data, pathological condition, diagnosis, treatment and prognosis of the disease of the patient.

In-patient Case Report	
Name:	Place of birth:
Sex:	Address:
Age:	Unit:
Nationality:	Time to be admitted (hour, month, day, year):
Marital status:	Time of data collecting (hour, month, day, year):
Occupation:	Teller of case history:
Solar terms when the disease occurred:	Reliability:

Chief complaint:
History of present illness:
Anamnesis:
Personal history:
Allergic history:
Obstetrical history:
Family history:

Physical Examination			
Temperature (T)	Pulse (P)	Respiration (R)	Blood pressure (BP)

Situation as a whole

Observation of vitality:

Observation of complexion:

Observation of appearance:

Observation of movement:

Sound:

Smell:

Tongue:

Pulse:

Superficial venule of index finger of an infant:

Skin, mucosa, lymph notes:

Mucocutaneous:

Lymph notes:

Head and face

Skull:

Eye:

Ear:

Nose:

Mouth cavity:

Neck

Shape:

Movement:

Trachea:

Thyroid:

Cervical vessels:

Chest

Thorax:

Breasts:

Lungs:

Heart:

Right (cm)	Intercostals space	Left (cm)
	II	
	III	
	IV	
	V	

Midclavicular line to median line is ___ cm

(including the results of inspection, palpation, percussion, and auscultation)

Peripheral vessels:

Abdomen

Liver:

Gall bladder:

Spleen:

Kidney:

Urinary bladder:

External urethral orifice and anus and excreta:

Spine and limbs

Spine:

Limbs:

Nails:

Nervous system

Superficial reflex:

Deep reflex:

Physiological reflex:

Pathologic reflex:

Others:

Meridians and points

Meridians:

Points:

Ear points:

(including the results of inspection, palpation, percussion, and auscultation)

Special examinations:

Laboratory examination:

Evidence of differentiation of disease and differentiation of syndrome:

Evidence of diagnosis of Western medicine:

Diagnosis on admission:

TCM diagnosis:

Diagnosis of disease:

Diagnosis of TCM syndrome:

Diagnosis of Western medicine:

Signature of resident:

Signature of visiting doctor:

In-patient Records	
Name:	Place of birth:
Sex:	Address:
Age:	Unit:
Nationality:	Time to be admitted (hour, day, month, year):
Marital status:	Time of data collecting (hour, day, month, year):
Occupation:	Teller of case history:
Solar terms when the disease occurred:	Reliability:

Chief complaint:

History of present illness:

Anamnesis:

Allergic history:

Others:

Physical Examination			
Temperature (T)	Pulse (P)	Respiration (R)	Blood pressure (BP)

Special examinations:

    Laboratory examination:

    Evidence of differentiation of disease and differentiation of syndrome:

    Evidence of diagnosis of Western medicine:

    Diagnosis on admission:

TCM diagnosis:

    Diagnosis of disease:

    Diagnosis of TCM syndrome:

Diagnosis of Western medicine:

         Signature of resident:

         Signature of visiting doctor:

GLOSSARY

Anuria   Failure of the kidneys to produce urine.

Aphtha   Small painful ulceration of the mouth.

Aphthous stomatitus   Inflammation of the soft tissue of the mouth, presenting with shallow painful ulcers.

Ascaris   A genus of the parasitic nematode worm.

Ascites   The accumulation of fluid in the peritoneal cavity, causing abdominal swelling.

Auricle   The flap of skin and cartilage that projects from the head at the exterior opening of the ear.

Blepharitis   Inflammation of the eyelids.

Buccal Mucosa   Mucous membrane in the mouth cavity.

Canthus   Either corner of the eye, where the eyelids meet.

Cardia   The opening of the oesophagus into the stomach.

Cellulitis   An infection of the deep dermis of the skin.

Desquamation   The removal of the outer layer of the epidermis of the skin by scaling.

Distal   Situated away from the point of attachment, or the median line of the body.

Dyspnoea   Laboured or difficult breathing.

Enuresis   The involuntary passing of urine.

Epigastric distention   Distention of the upper central region of the abdomen.

Epigastrium   The upper central region of the abdomen.

Epiglottis   Thin flap of cartilage behind the tongue that covers the entrance to the larynx when swallowing.

Epistaxis   A nosebleed.

Erysipelas   Infection of the skin, characterized by redness and swelling.

Exophthalmos   Unusual protrusion of the eyeballs in their sockets.

Fistula   An abnormal passage between two hollow organs, or between an organ and the exterior of the body.

Furuncles   Inflamed area of the skin containing pus, otherwise known as a boil.

Gastroptosis   A condition in which the stomach hangs low in the abdomen.

Glabellum   The flat area of the skull between the eyebrows.

Glaucoma   The loss of vision due to damage caused by abnormally high pressure in the eye.

Goitre   Swelling of the neck due to enlargement of the thyroid gland.

Haematemisis   The vomiting of blood.

Hemiplegia   Paralysis of one side of the body.

Haematochezia   The passing of blood from the anus.

Haemoptysis   The coughing up of blood; or blood stained sputum.

Heterotropia   A squint, or abnormal alignment of the eyes.

Hypochondriac distention   Distention of the upper lateral portion of the abdomen, situated behind the lower ribs.

Ileocecal conjunction   The point at which the large and small intestines connect.

Jaundice   A yellowing of the skin or the whites of the eyes.

Kyphosis   The outward curvature of the spine, if excessive causes hunching of the back.

Lepra   Leprosy, a chronic disease that affects skin, mucous membranes and nerves.

Leucorrhoea   A thick whitish or yellowish vaginal discharge.

Lochiorrhea   Profuse flow of the lochia, the vaginal discharge following childbirth.

Macrocrania   The abnormal increase of the size of the skull in relation to the face.

Macule   A flat discoloured area on the skin.

Meatus   A passage or opening, such as the auditory meatus from the outer ear to the ear drum.

Metopism   The persistence into adulthood of the suture between the frontal plates of the skull.

Microcrania   The abnormal decrease of the size of the skull in relation to the face.

Miliaria alba   An itchy heat rash with small white crystal like granules raised above the skin.

Mydriasis   Prolonged abnormal dilation of the eye.

Oedema   The swelling of soft tissue due to excess water accumulation.

Opisthotonus   The position of the body in which the head, neck and spine are arched backwards.

Papilla   A small nipple like projection.

Parasitosis   Infestation or infection with parasites.

Polyp   A growth protruding from a mucous membrane.

Prospermia   Premature ejaculation.

Proximal   Situated close to the point of attachment, or the median line of the body.

Ptosis   Drooping of the upper eyelid.

Pylorus   The passage that connects the stomach and the duodenum.

Rhinorrhoea   Excessive mucous secretion from the nose.

Rosacea   A chronic inflammatory skin disease in which the skin is abnormally flushed.

Scrofula   A tuberculosis infection of the skin, usually in the neck.

Tenesmus   The frequent or constant sensation of the need to defecate without the production of significant quantities of faeces.

Thorax   The part of the body between the neck and the diaphragm.

Tympanites   Distention of the stomach with air or gas.

Varicella   Commonly known as chickenpox, a highly infectious disease transmitted by airborne droplets.

Venous   Relating to the veins.

BIBLIOGRAPHY

Huang Di Nei Jing Su Wen (1979) 'Plain Questions.' *The Yellow Emperor's Classic of Internal Medicine*. Beijing: People's Health Publishing House.

Huang Di Nei Jing Ling Shu (1979) 'Miraculous Pivot.' *The Yellow Emperor's Classic of Internal Medicine*. Beijing: People's Health Publishing House.

Huang-fu Mi (1979) *Systematic Classic of Acupuncture and Moxibustio*n. Bejing: People's Press.

Zhang Zhong Jing (2007) *Treatise on Febrile Diseases*. Translated by Luo Xiwen. Canada: Redwing Book Company.

INDEX